Updates in Surgery

The aim of this series is to provide informative updates on hot topics in the areas of breast, endocrine, and abdominal surgery, surgical oncology, and coloproctology, and on new surgical techniques such as robotic surgery, laparoscopy, and minimally invasive surgery. Readers will find detailed guidance on patient selection, performance of surgical procedures, and avoidance of complications. In addition, a range of other important aspects are covered, from the role of new imaging tools to the use of combined treatments and postoperative care.

The topics addressed by volumes in the series Updates in Surgery have been selected for their broad significance in collaboration with the Italian Society of Surgery. Each volume will assist surgical residents and fellows and practicing surgeons in reaching appropriate treatment decisions and achieving optimal outcomes. The series will also be highly relevant for surgical researchers.

Paolo Carcoforo • Fausto Catena
Editors

Geriatric Surgery

Springer

Editors
Paolo Carcoforo
Breast Surgery Unit
Ferrara University Hospital
Cona, Ferrara, Italy

Fausto Catena
Department of Medical and Surgical Sciences
Alma Mater Studiorum
University of Bologna
Bologna, Italy

ISSN 2280-9848 ISSN 2281-0854 (electronic)
Updates in Surgery
ISBN 978-3-032-24280-8 ISBN 978-3-032-24281-5 (eBook)
https://doi.org/10.1007/978-3-032-24281-5

This work was supported by Italian Society of Surgery.

This Springer imprint is published by the registered company Springer Nature Switzerland AG
The registered company address is: Gewerbestrasse 11, 6330 Cham, Switzerland

Foreword

It is with sincere satisfaction that I present the work of Paolo Carcoforo and Fausto Catena, published as the Biennial Report of the Italian Society of Surgery on the topic of geriatric surgery.

This volume is comprehensive and of outstanding academic quality, bringing together clinical experience, theoretical reflections, and methodological updates: "between history and the future: passion, empathy, expertise, and artificial intelligence." It represents a mature synthesis of surgical tradition and innovation, highlighting the increasingly central role of the management of older patients in contemporary clinical practice.

The work opens with a historical overview of the development of geriatric surgery in Italy, rigorously reconstructing the cultural and institutional pathway that led to the emergence and establishment of this discipline. From the trailblazing phase—characterized by a predominantly emergency-based approach and by the perception of the elderly patient as a "high-risk" subject—the field has progressively evolved toward an organized model based on patient selection criteria, surgical planning, and multidimensional assessment.

The fundamental principles of the discipline are developed by placing the biological complexity of aging at the center of the analysis, emphasizing the distinction between chronological and biological age, together with the progressive decline in organ functional reserve, which determines a distinctive vulnerability to surgical stress. The work also provides an extensive analysis of surgical risk and perioperative management.

Drawing on their extensive experience, the authors emphasize the need for risk stratification models integrating comorbidities, functional status, and frailty, thereby overcoming the limitations of traditional models and framing surgical decision-making as a complex and individualized process. The issue of informed consent is also thoroughly addressed, with particular emphasis on the appropriateness of surgical indications, which must necessarily be weighed against the expected quality of life.

The volume highlights the role of integrated care, underscoring the importance of nursing support and home care services, while outlining innovative organizational models focused on continuity of care. Another distinctive strength of the work lies in its analysis of enhanced recovery protocols, including Fast-Track and ERAS programs, demonstrating how adaptation of these strategies to the elderly population can significantly reduce complications, hospital length of stay, and postoperative functional decline.

The volume also stands out for the breadth of its specialist coverage, with dedicated contributions addressing the various surgical subspecialties. It examines the specific features of breast surgery in older patients, discusses the challenges of thyroid and parathyroid surgery, and explores pancreatic surgery as well as surgery for chronic inflammatory bowel diseases, highlighting the critical issues related to patient selection and management of potential complications. Particularly noteworthy are the contributions on full-thickness rectal prolapse and emergency surgery in the elderly, clinical settings in which operative risk reaches its highest levels and requires rapid yet carefully balanced decision-making.

Technological innovation is explored in the chapters devoted to robotic surgery and day surgery, which open new perspectives for selected geriatric patients in terms of minimally invasive approaches and reduction of the physiological impact of surgery. The work also provides extensive coverage of digestive tract oncologic surgery, including esophagogastric, colorectal, hepatobiliary, and abdominal wall surgery. Across all these fields, the decisive role of patient selection, minimally invasive techniques, and personalized treatment strategies clearly emerges. The volume concludes with a contribution on bariatric surgery in the elderly patient, an increasingly relevant topic that poses new challenges in terms of indications, safety, and efficacy.

Finally, the discussion of future perspectives is of great significance, particularly regarding the application of artificial intelligence in predictive risk models, precision medicine, and the development of dedicated care pathways. At the same time, an ethical reflection emerges, emphasizing the need to keep the individual, in his or her entirety, at the center of the decision-making process.

Overall, this collection represents a scientific contribution of outstanding value, capable of integrating methodological rigor, clinical expertise, and forward-looking vision. It stands as an authoritative reference for surgeons and geriatricians, offering both conceptual and practical tools to address competently and responsibly the challenges posed by the aging surgical population, in keeping with the principles of an increasingly personalized and multidisciplinary medicine.

President of the Italian Society of Surgery — Ludovico Docimo
Naples, Italy
September 2026

Preface

Geriatric surgery is a cross-disciplinary specialty that encompasses all fields of surgery.

The geriatric population is rapidly increasing in high-income countries and now represents the group undergoing the majority of surgical procedures. Elderly patients present unique characteristics related to their intrinsic frailty. It is therefore reasonable to expect that, much like pediatric surgery, geriatric surgery will become the specialty of the future, acting as a unifying bridge among the various subspecialties into which general surgery has currently evolved.

This book aims to support the surgical care of elderly patients across different subspecialty areas. We strongly believe that readers will benefit from this renewed, holistic vision of general surgery as an integrated discipline, as it once was in the past.

We thank the Italian Society of Surgery for granting us this privilege and opportunity, and the Italian Society of Surgical Physiopathology for the collaboration in developing the project.

Ferrara, Italy
Bologna, Italy
September 2026

Paolo Carcoforo
Fausto Catena

Contents

Italian Society of Geriatric Surgery: A Historical Overview

1

Oreste Terranova

The Italian Society of Geriatric Surgery (SICG) was founded in Naples in 1986 on the initiative of Prof. Giuseppe Negro, Professor of Surgery at the University of that city. However, the story begins several years earlier with repeated contacts between Negro and Prof. Oreste Terranova from the University of Padua. At the end of the 1970s, this university temporarily hosted the Italian Society of Gerontology and Geriatrics, chaired by Prof. Gaetano Crepaldi, Professor of Geriatrics. This society brought together nearly all Italian geriatricians—university-based, hospital-employed, and in the community—and was very active across Italy through numerous academic and public initiatives aimed at raising awareness among politicians and society regarding elderly issues.

In Padua, thanks also to the sensitivity of Dr. Pietro Terranova, Medical Director of the National Institute for Insurance against Diseases, and the Department of Social Services of the Municipality of Padua, the society managed to establish an agreement with these institutions to provide free at-home specialist geriatrician care.

This intense activity and the results achieved led Negro and Terranova to contact Crepaldi in order to involve surgeons interested in elderly patients within the Society of Gerontology. Their goal was to raise awareness in the academic and hospital worlds about the surgical problems related to elderly patients.

Until then, elderly patients were typically only operated on when absolutely necessary. Surgeries were performed almost exclusively in emergency settings, when the patient was already considered nearly beyond help—hence, surgery was a last resort. Elective surgery was very rare.

Surgical risk was almost always deemed extremely high, and alternative treatments (even if ineffective) or no treatment at all were usually preferred. When a surgeon deemed the risk low enough, or if the patient or their relatives insisted on

O. Terranova (✉)
General Surgery, Padua University, Padua, Italy
e-mail: oreste.terranova@unipd.it

P. Carcoforo, F. Catena (eds.), *Geriatric Surgery*, Updates in Surgery,
https://doi.org/10.1007/978-3-032-24281-5_1

surgery, it was always performed by the institute's director, who was certainly the best diagnostician, quickest at intraoperative decisions, and most technically skilled.

Preoperative diagnostics were very limited—ultrasound, CT, MRI and similar tools did not exist. Often, the diagnosis had to be made during surgery. Once a diagnosis was made, the most appropriate surgical solution had to be chosen. Anesthesia, especially if prolonged, was considered a major postoperative risk. Therefore, when operating on elderly patients, the surgeon had to be highly experienced, well versed in various surgical techniques, confident, and quick. Complications were to be avoided at all costs because in elderly patients they significantly increased surgical risk. This remains true today.

Complications often led to bed rest, which increased the likelihood of pressure ulcers and serious respiratory and cardiac problems. Recovery, which was already slow in a "regular" postoperative course, could become extremely lengthy—or even absent—leading to death.

Gerontology showed great interest in the surgeons' objectives, and Negro and Terranova were elected to the Society's Executive Committee. Annual society congresses began to include a dedicated space for geriatric surgery. This collaboration continued until 1986, when the decision was made to become "independent". Negro gathered 17 colleagues in Naples (Alessandro Agresti, Giovanni Arciero, Francesco Battocchio, Vanni Beltrami, Giancarlo Botta, Francesco Crucitti, Davide D'Amico, Mario Fersini, Francesco Lo Schiavo, Alberto Montori, Anacleto Peracchia, Vittorio Piegari, Giovanni Persico, Sergio Tartaro, Oreste Terranova, Giampaolo Zelli) and proposed the creation of an association named Italian Society of Geriatric Surgery.

Relations with the Society of Gerontology remained characterized by a spirit of collaboration and collegiality and continue to this day.

The presidency of the society has been held by several prominent figures in Italian surgery. Chronologically, from 1986 to 2001: Antonio Rodolico, Anacleto Peracchia, Vittorio Piegari, Vincenzo Martinelli, Beniamino Tesauro, Piero Pietri, Vanni Beltrami, Oreste Terranova, Paolo Melita, Luigi Roncoroni. More recently: Francesco Sciannameo, Giovanni Persico, Mario Nano, Silvio Canonico, Francesco Basile, Francesco Gabrielli, Alessandro Puzziello, Nicola Avenia, Paolo Carcoforo.

There has always been great enthusiasm and prestige surrounding the society. Many board members made important contributions, especially in the early years, helping to establish the society by organizing congresses, conferences, training courses, and promoting the inclusion of geriatric surgery in medical school curricula and specialization programs. They also encouraged the establishment of geriatric surgery wards in university hospitals and general hospitals (Naples, Padua, Turin, Rome, Catania, Messina, Ancona).

In Padua—unique in Italy—a joint university-hospital Department of Elderly Care was established, led by a geriatric surgeon. It included the Geriatrics and Geriatric Surgery divisions, Geriatrics 1 and 2, Long-Term Care Units 1 and 2, as well as physical therapy, psychology, rehabilitation, and social services.

Among the many dedicated colleagues, notable names following the order of board membership include: Giampaolo Zelli from Rome, Alberto Montori from Rome, Francesco Campana from Rome, Martino Bonomo from Bari, Luigi Moggi from Perugia, Natalino Guernelli from Bologna, Gastone Veroux from Catania, Nino Masera from Turin, Aldo Leggeri from Trieste, Giorgio Bucciarelli from Florence, Vincenzo Di Giovanni from Rome, Vittorio Sommariva from Palermo, Alfonso Pannella from Pavia, Tommaso Mercadante from Palermo, Antonino Giovinetto from Catania, Ercole Cirino from Catania, Gianfranco Azzena from Ferrara, Ettore Masenti from Turin, Achille Tarquini from Cagliari, Vincenzo Violi from Parma, Raffaele Jovino from Naples, Giacomo Bajamonte from Palermo, Napoleone Massaioli from Turin, Mauro Roseano from Trieste, Costante Natale from Foggia.

A special mention goes to Mario Nano from Turin, who joined the board in 1994 and became president in 2010, and to Francesco Gabrielli from Milan, a board member since 1997 and president in 2018, for their ongoing, dedicated, and constructive commitment to the society.

Another heartfelt memory goes to Francesco Battocchio, founding member and father of Piero (currently a board member), who was instrumental in organizing the third society congress in Padua and advocating for the rights of elderly patients. Few people could connect with the elderly as he did—with gentleness, kindness, and a smile, combined with surgical skills well above the norm. Sadly, he passed away prematurely.

By 2001, the SICG membership was second in number only to the Italian Society of Surgery (SIC). In Padua, with major contributions from Bruno Martella and Carmelo Militello, the Society's biannual Bulletin was published for a decade (1990–2000). Subsequently, the SIC referred to the prestigious journal *Il Giornale di Chirurgia*, directed by Prof. G. Di Matteo, a renowned surgeon and academic.

The first congress was held in Naples in 1987 with Giuseppe Negro, followed by the second in Palermo (1988) with Prof. Nino Rodolico, the third in Padua with Oreste Terranova, continuing through to 2019 in Genoa. Memorable annual meetings took place in Parma (Anacleto Peracchia), Perugia (Luigi Moggi), Naples (Vittorio Piegari), Rome (Vincenzo Martinelli), Turin (Ettore Masenti), Milan (Piero Pietri), Chieti (Giacomo Gidaro), Trieste (Aldo Leggeri), Padua (Oreste Terranova), Messina (Paolo Melita), Parma (Luigi Roncoroni), Terni (Francesco Sciannameo), Catanzaro (Stefano De Franciscis), Turin (Mario Nano), Naples (Silvio Canonico and Giovanni Persico), Catania (Francesco Basile), Rome (Antonio Crucitti), and Lecce (Andrea Renda).

Since 2018, every other year, the SICG National Congress has merged in Rome with the joint event of the SIC. Even during the COVID pandemic, under the presidency of Alessandro Puzziello and Nicola Avenia, the Society's scientific and educational activities continued through webinars and remote meetings.

In 2012, Padua hosted the 25th Congress during the "Week of the Elderly", organized with many city-wide and regional events by the inter-institutional Department of Elderly Care. The goal was to raise public awareness of elderly issues by involving the university, local institutions, volunteers, schools, care homes, media, and healthcare providers. This initiative embodied the mission of SICG: placing the well-being of the elderly at the center of its efforts.

Through its congresses and training, SICG has always conveyed to students and residents that elderly patients are "special patients" who require equally special care. Every patient enters the hospital with trepidation—but especially the elderly, who suddenly realize their own fragility. They fear not returning home, the anesthesia, the surgery, and losing autonomy. Even if they continue to smile, these thoughts are always present.

The surgeon must listen with patience and humanity, explain the condition clearly and sensitively, and share how they plan to address the situation. During surgery, the focus should be on techniques that truly benefit the patient—not on showcasing surgical prowess. Postoperative mobilization should begin as early as possible, not only to prevent complications from bed rest but to give the patient confidence in recovery and moving beyond the most delicate phase. Communication between surgeon and patient must be immediate, human, and never rushed.

In 1982 in Turin, 4 years before the founding of SICG, another pioneer in geriatric surgery, Prof. Nino Masera, established the "Masera-Biancalana Foundation for Operated Elderly Patients" (now the Nino Masera Foundation). Their research focused on surgical risk and the postoperative life of elderly patients. The Foundation has regional branches and awards scholarships to deserving students.

Masera moved to Ancona to direct the National Institute for Rest and Care of the Elderly (INRCA—IRCCS), the only public scientific research hospital dedicated specifically to gerontology and geriatrics. The Foundation also relocated to Ancona. Masera joined the SICG board in 1989, and with his involvement, the so-called "historic group" of Italian geriatric surgeons was formed (Giuseppe Negro, Vittorio Piegari, Nino Masera, Oreste Terranova). They aimed to promote elderly surgery at the European level, and in December 1989, the "Société Européenne de Chirurgie Gériatrique" was founded in Paris. Founding members included M. Bussone (France), S. El Banna (Belgium), O. Gagey (France), P. Hoffmeyer (Switzerland), P. Mendes Da Costa (Belgium), G. Negro, and O. Terranova. The first president was Michel Bussone, with Giuseppe Negro as vice-president and Pierre Mendes Da Costa as secretary-general.

The society later expanded to include British and Scottish colleagues, holding biennial congresses from 1995 to 2012, alternating between Paris (organized by Bussone) and Padua (organized by Terranova). It has not convened since 2012.

The vitality of our society, since its founding, has been rooted in the friendships between colleagues, mutual respect, scientific collaboration, and deep concern for elderly patients. After almost 40 years, the society is more alive and stronger than ever. President Francesco Gabrielli, assisted by the tireless and dynamic secretary general Bruno Amato of the University of Naples, has revitalized the society admirably—completing the relationship with Federanziani, gaining accreditation with the Ministry of Health, and continuing to support regional congresses (Padua, Reggio Emilia, Turin, Salerno). After him, Puzziello, Avenia, and Carcoforo continued—and continue—to carry forward equally important initiatives in scientific research and continuing education.

Certainly, new technologies and equipment have transformed our field, but the elderly patient remains that special individual we all know. So when we are in front of them and their illness, let us always remember that we are dealing with a human being—not a machine to be overhauled.

2 Principles of Geriatric Surgery

Mario Nano and Mario Solej

2.1 Introduction

Geriatric surgery is the branch of medicine concerned with the surgical care of older adults. To meet the special needs of these patients and restore the highest possible level of practical functioning, it applies the principles of general surgery coupled with the formal assessment of potential risks and benefits, treatment options and outcomes. Because preservation of functional independence is considered a more meaningful patient-reported endpoint than disease-free survival, determining the factors that can predict the maintenance of functional status is of critical importance in health care delivery to the elderly [1–4].

Broadly defined, aging is a complex, differentiated process. Age-related biological parameters diverge as people grow older, whereas they tend to converge toward a narrower range of mean values in the young. Moreover, the trajectory of functional decline is malleable and can be reversed in many organs and systems. In living organisms, aging is a physiological, genetically programmed, universal, and heterochronic process. The term "heterochronic" describes the phenomenon that organs and systems senesce at different rates in the same organism. Heterochronic senescence is of central importance to geriatric medicine and surgery for distinguishing between diseases (curable or treatable) and incurable heterochronic conditions. For example, a 70-year-old with diabetes has a condition that a physician can treat. Conversely, a 70-year-old afflicted with panvasculopathy has a heterochronic

M. Nano (✉)
Fellow of the American College of Surgeons, General Surgery, San Luigi Gonzaga Hospital, University of Turin, Orbassano, TO, Italy
e-mail: marionano.md@gmail.com

M. Solej
SCDU General Surgery, San Luigi Gonzaga Hospital, Orbassano, TO, Italy

P. Carcoforo, F. Catena (eds.), *Geriatric Surgery*, Updates in Surgery,
https://doi.org/10.1007/978-3-032-24281-5_2

condition in which the cardiovascular system shows clinical signs about which the physician can do nothing.

Another aspect of aging is the difference between normality and normal: normality refers to physiological function in relation to biological age; normal is a statistical concept that refers to levels of functioning according to age class. To illustrate, arthrosis in an 80-year-old can be regarded as "normal" because it occurs statistically in many patients; however, it is not the normality since joint aging does not lead to severe cartilage deterioration. In fact, not all older adults suffer from arthrosis. Whereas normality refers to a physiological-functional condition, and hence is an objective fact, normal refers to a subjective evaluation of functioning along a spectrum of cultural norms and social compliance. A 90-year-old woman with urinary incontinence, but otherwise self-sufficient and cognitively oriented, would be regarded by her family as being "normal" but not by nursing home administrators since her condition would mean extra work for the facility staff.

A third distinction to be made in aging concerns the difference between physiological condition and pathological condition. While the boundary between the two is usually clear in younger patients, it is blurred in the elderly and is more of a qualitative than a quantitative nature. This leads to a discussion of the differences between chronological age and biological age.

Aging is characterized by homeostasis: a functional older adult may maintain good health into old age but will become increasingly vulnerable to stress and illness as physiological reserve decreases [5, 6]. The difference between chronological age and biological age derives from the difference between the functional reserve statistically expected for a given age group and the physiological reserve an individual patient actually has. Over the past century, the average life expectancy has increased and with it a *life span beyond age* 80 is now more common in Europe and the United States. At this stage of older age, an elderly person's sociofunctional status can be classified from fit to frail (fit, pre-frail, frail).

In older adults, the surgical management of diseases is often complicated by age-related physiological changes and altered response to treatment. Besides prolonged hospitalization and bed rest, other factors including immobilization, reduced plasma volume, sensory deprivation, and reduced dietary intake can deplete the patient's physiologic reserve, precipitating further functional decline or irreversible dependence. Biological age, which is the cumulative result of pathophysiological aging, comorbidity, and genetic factors, seems to be a better predictor of the degree of fitness and performance status of a patient during an illness [5].

For this reason, geriatrics (medical and surgical) embraces a holistic approach rather than the disease-based model of conventional medicine. Consistent with this holistic view is the notion that there are no "elderly diseases" (like there are childhood diseases), but that certain diseases occur more often in older age. Central to geriatrics is the assessment of how an older adult's organism reacts to a disease, which will differ from that of a younger adult. In geriatric surgery, successful patient outcome is not the result of surgical technique but rather of a deep understanding of the geriatric patient.

In the surgical care of older patients, several factors increase susceptibility to perioperative stress:

- Low physiological reserve
- Slow recovery rate
- Difficult adaptation
- Increased susceptibility to bleeding, hypotension, hypovolemia, anoxia
- Increased susceptibility to constipation and meteorism
- Lower resistance to infections
- Increased susceptibility to intravasal coagulation
- More catabolic metabolism
- Hypoventilation due to rigid rib cage and weak diaphragm.

These factors categorize the older adult as a high-risk surgical patient. Based on personal experience [7], 25% of risk is attributable to age and surgical disease, while the general condition of body systems needed to respond to surgical stress accounts for the remaining 75%. To illustrate this point, we can take as an example a risk calculation model for a patient with diabetes [8]. The model uses a simple equation for calculating biological age: chronological age plus duration of diabetes in years. For instance, a 65-year-old with a 10-year history of diabetes presents the same clinical problems as those statistically expected for a 75-year-old. Surgical treatment of a diabetic patient involves not only glycemic control but also management of the risks associated with the systemic complications of diabetes. Because of the age-related decline in organ and system function, older age constitutes a surgical risk factor *per se*: the older the patient, the lower the functional reserve, the higher the surgical risk irrespective of associated pathologies.

"The traditional view in surgical and clinical care is that age does not matter when survival outcomes involve the oldest-old patients". This notion has been challenged by strong evidence to the contrary. Because the aging process diminishes the physiological functional reserve of vital organs, chronological age in itself constitutes an established risk factor [3, 9]. This is, in fact, substantiated by the observation of a decline in renal function (slower glomerular filtration rate, decreased ability to concentrate and dilute urine), cardiocirculatory function (lower maximal heart rate, decreased myocardial and vascular adrenergic response), and respiratory function (reduced elastic lung recoil and closing volume, altered ventilation/perfusion ratio with increased intrapulmonary shunt). Since these changes can affect the entire geriatric population, advanced age represents a surgical risk and poses both the patient and the surgical care team with difficult decisions about major surgery.

In geriatric surgery, risk assessment is of fundamental importance. Several models for the assessment of surgical risk in the elderly have been developed, some of which involving complex mathematical calculations [10]. Despite its limitations, the American Society of Anesthesiologists (ASA) Physical Status classification system, initially created in 1941 and revised several times since then, is the simplest and most practical grading system currently available to evaluate a patient's preoperative physical state and surgical risk also in geriatric patients. When coupled with the Comprehensive Geriatric Assessment (CGA) scheme, it can be used to assess various physical, social, and psychosocial dimensions in the elderly. Other classification systems, such as the Reiss Index [11, 12], also investigate these variables. A simple arithmetic calculation is insufficient to predict surgical risk in such complex patients, however. Treatment options need to be personalized and based on a deep understanding of geriatrics. "An expert opinion would be required at the bedside. Scoring will never replace clinical judgment" [13].

Where geriatric medicine and surgery differ from other branches of medicine is the extent to which a patient's medical history, epidemiology of diseases, presence of coexisting conditions, need for functional assessment, decompensation cascade, drug therapy, and real-life circumstances all come into play in the delivery of care. One of the principal challenges of clinical geriatrics is early diagnosis owing to the difficulty in obtaining a history and the problems with interpreting symptoms [14].

Interpreting symptoms is challenging, particularly so in older adults. A helpful mnemonic is the triad: altered signs and symptoms, masked signs and symptoms, and variable signs and symptoms.

- Altered signs and symptoms. Pain symptoms may be attenuated or absent (silent suffering of organ systems). Because signs of peritonism may be vague, and hyperthermia and leukocytosis limited to the acute event (e.g., diverticular perforation), the event may go unrecognized, resulting in delayed diagnosis and hospitalization for an advanced stage of generalized peritonitis. There are other associated diseases which, if complicated, can mimic a surgical disease. For example, metabolic acidosis in a diabetic patient can resemble acute surgical abdomen manifesting with abdominal pain, rebound tenderness (positive Blumberg sign), vomiting, fever, cutaneous hyperesthesia, and leukocytosis. Establishing the differential diagnosis between diabetic ketoacidosis-induced false acute abdomen and true acute surgical abdomen is complicated by ketoacidosis. A useful clue in diagnosis of the former is that pain is preceded by nausea, vomiting, and polydipsia.
- Masked signs and symptoms. The presence of coexisting conditions further complicates interpreting symptoms. In addition, an acute event may precipitate a coexisting illness, distracting attention away from the acute event and delaying diagnosis. For example, in a patient with heart disease, an initially oligosymptomatic peritonitis may be the cause of an episode of congestive heart failure, drawing clinical attention only to the acute event.
- Variable signs and symptoms. There are certain diseases that can manifest very differently from those typically seen in younger patients. Hyperthyroidism can manifest with the classic symptoms of hypothyroidism (apathetic hyperthyroidism), making it difficult to establish the clinical diagnosis in relation to senile involutional cerebropathy.

2.2 Frailty

The term "frailty" in reference to the elderly describes a range of conditions in older people, including general debility, cognitive impairment, and living in a structurally and socially marginalized environment [15].

Frailty encompasses socioeconomic, psychological, health care, and biological aspects, any one of which may predominate in an individual older person, though there is a common denominator. Largely ignored by conventional medicine, the frail elderly are considered scientifically uninteresting, ungratifying professionally, unhealable, troublesome to manage, costly, and difficult to discharge [16]. The prevention, identification, and treatment of frailty are the core concern and main challenge in modern geriatric medicine [17, 18].

The general profile of the frail elderly patient is characterized by advanced or very advanced age, multiple chronic illnesses, disability, socioeconomic problems, loneliness and poverty, and precarious homeostasis due to multisystem failure that trigger the so-called "failure cascade" associated with elevated mortality. Added to these conditions are biological and biochemical abnormalities of uncertain origin that are the hallmarks of frailty: elevated C-reactive protein (CRP), interleukin-6 (IL-6), tumor necrosis factor-α (TNF-α), D-dimer, osteopenia, sarcopenia, anemia, insulin resistance, and decreased iron, vitamin B12, folate, and albumin levels [19, 20].

In 1976 Bernard Isaac described the "four giants of geriatrics" – incontinence, immobility, instability (falls), and intellectual impairment – from which five geriatric syndromes were subsequently derived: pressure ulcers, incontinence, falls, functional decline, and delirium [21, 22]. The frail elderly patient is categorized as such when three of these five syndromes are present.

Frailty is a dynamic condition that can be measured. The two major models for the assessment of frailty are the Frailty Phenotype, devised by Fried and coworkers [18], and the Frailty Index proposed by Rockwood and colleagues [23]. The Frailty Phenotype (FP) is based on the assessment of five parameters [24]:

1. Unintentional weight loss over the past year (10 lbs. or 4.5 kg)
2. Self-reported exhaustion on at least 3 days/week
3. Reduced muscle strength as evaluated by hand grip (less than 13 lbs. or 5.85 kg for men and 7.5 lbs. or 3.37 kg for women)
4. Reduced physical activity as measured with the Physical Activity Scale for the Elderly (PASE)
5. Reduced gait speed over a known distance (more than 7 seconds to cover 4.57 m).

If three of these five features are present, the patient is deemed as frail; if one to two are present, the patient is categorized as pre-frail; if none are present the patient is considered fit.

The Frailty Index (FI) conceptualizes frailty as a syndrome characterized by the loss of physiological reserve due to the accumulation of deficits, resulting in vulnerability to stress. The Index is derived from the Canadian Study of Heath and Aging (CSHA) and comprises 70 items. It is calculated by dividing the number of deficits in a patient by the number of deficits measured [25, 26]. The Index is composed of five scores: 0 (no positive items), 0.33 (1/4 positive items), 0.67 (3/4 positive items), 1 (all positive items – indicating maximum severity of frailty).

However, neither of these assessment tools takes into account many of the other important factors that contribute to frailty, such as living alone, social engagement, empowerment/life control, and socioeconomic status. The best instrument for assessing frailty is the Comprehensive Geriatric Assessment (CGA) defined as a multidimensional diagnostic process intended to determine an older person's medical, physicosocial, and functional limitations. Among the many assessment scales described in the literature, the most widely used are the Clinical Frailty Scale (CFS), the Growing Frailty Indicator (GFI), the Tilburg Frail Indicator (TFI), and the Edmonton Frailty Scale (EFS) [27].

Since more and more older patients with comorbidities undergo surgery [28], surgeons have begun to use frailty as a predictive tool to identify those at risk for poor outcomes [22, 29, 30]. In patients over age 75 years, frailty is associated with increased postoperative mortality, postoperative complications, prolonged hospital stay, discharge to residential care, unplanned three-month readmission, increased three-month mortality, and a three- to eight-fold higher incidence of postoperative delirium in elective and emergency abdominal surgery [21, 31–33]. The CGA has been shown to predict postoperative complications in frail elderly patients better than chronological age predicts postoperative mortality [34]. Unfortunately, none of these three tools (CGA, FI, FP) has been adopted in routine preoperative assessment. The CGA is the most comprehensive, while the FP is the simplest. Although the FP measures only physical performance, it may provide a valid clinical tool and starting point for the assessment of frailty in surgical patients [35].

Acknowledgments The current chapter is an update of the homonymous one, published in the volume Surgical Management of Elderly Patients (Springer, 2018, A. Crucitti ed.) and authored by Mario Nano and Mario Solej.

References

1. Ugolini G, Pasini F, Ghignone F, et al. How to select elderly colorectal cancer patients for surgery: a pilot study in an Italian academic medical center. Cancer Biol Med. 2015;12(4):302–7.
2. PACE participants, Audisio RA, Pope D, et al. Shall we operate? Preoperative assessment in elderly cancer patients (PACE) can help. A SIOG surgical task force prospective study. Crit Rev Oncol Hematol. 2008;65(2):156–63.
3. Kim YW, Kim IY. Factors associated with postoperative complications and 1-year mortality after surgery for colorectal cancer in octogenarians and nonagenarians. Clin Interv Aging. 2016;11:689–97.
4. Hamel MB, Henderson WG, Khuri SF, Daley J. Surgical outcomes for patients aged 80 and older: morbidity and mortality from major noncardiac surgery. J Am Geriatr Soc. 2005;53(3):424–9.

5. Dewan SK, Zheng SB, Xia SJ. Preoperative geriatric assessment: comprehensive, multidisciplinary and proactive. Eur J Intern Med. 2012;23(6):487–94.
6. Feng MA, McMillan DT, Crowell K, et al. Geriatric assessment in surgical oncology: a systematic review. J Surg Res. 2015;193(1):265–72.
7. Masera N. Principi e fondamentali della chirurgia geriatrica. In: Masera N, Ferrara L, Nano M, editors. Chirurgia geriatrica. Torino: Minerva Medica; 1990.
8. Fumelli P. Chirurgia e diabete senile. In: Masera N, Ferrara L, Nano M, editors. Chirurgia geriatrica. Torino: Minerva Medica; 1990.
9. Chung JY, Chang WY, Lin TW, et al. An analysis of surgical outcomes in patients aged 80 years and older. Acta Anaesthesiol Taiwanica. 2014;52(4):153–8.
10. Nano M. Problemi chirurgici. In: Tammaro AE, Casale G, Frustaglia A, editors. Manuale di geriatria e gerontologia. Milano: McGraw-Hill; 1996.
11. Leardi S, De Santis C, Ciuca B, et al. Risk indices in geriatric surgery: ASA index versus Reiss index. Minerva Chir. 1997;52(3):255–60. Italian.
12. Reiss R, Deutsch AA, Nudelman I, Gutman H. Multifactorial analysis of prognostic factors in emergency abdominal surgery in patients above 80 years. Analysis of 154 consecutive cases. Int Surg. 1989;74(2):93–6.
13. Marchionni N, Moschi G, Di Bari M, et al. Acute and long-term effects of flosequinan in patients with chronic cardiac failure. Am Heart J. 1993;126(1):147–54.
14. Katlic MR. Principles of geriatric surgery. In: Rosenthal RA, Zenilman ME, Katlic MR, editors. Principles and practice of geriatric surgery. 2nd ed. New York: Springer; 2011.
15. Ruggiero C, Cherubini A, Senin U. Alla scoperta delle origini dell'anziano fragile. G Gerontol. 2007;55:183–90.
16. Makary MA, Segev DL, Pronovost PJ, et al. Frailty as a predictor of surgical outcomes in older patients. J Am Coll Surg. 2010;210(6):901–8.
17. Pilotto A, Ferrucci L. Verso una definizione clinica della fragilità: utilità dell'approccio multidimensionale. G Gerontol. 2011;59:125–9.
18. Fried LP, Tangen CM, Walston J, et al. Frailty in older adults: evidence for a phenotype. J Gerontol A Biol Sci Med Sci. 2001;56(3):M146–56.
19. Orandi BJ, Winter JM, Segev DL, Makary MA. Frailty and surgery in the elderly. In: Rosenthal RA, Zenilman ME, Katlic MR, editors. Principles and practice of geriatric surgery. 2nd ed. New York: Springer; 2011.
20. Partridge JS, Harari D, Dhesi JK. Frailty in the older surgical patient: a review. Age Ageing. 2012;41(2):142–7.
21. Jones TS, Dunn CL, Wu DS, et al. Relationship between asking an older adult about falls and surgical outcomes. JAMA Surg. 2013;148(12):1132–8.
22. Robinson TN, Eiseman B, Wallace JI, et al. Redefining geriatric preoperative assessment using frailty, disability and co-morbidity. Ann Surg. 2009;250(3):449–55.
23. Rockwood K, Song X, MacKnight C, et al. A global clinical measure of fitness and frailty in elderly people. CMAJ. 2005;173(5):489–95.
24. Foroni M, Mussi C, Erzili E, Salvioli G. L'anziano fragile e il paziente anziano fragile: problema solo terminologico? G Gerontol. 2006;54:255–9.
25. Fagard K, Leonard S, Deschodt M, et al. The impact of frailty on postoperative outcomes in individuals aged 65 and over undergoing elective surgery for colorectal cancer: a systematic review. J Geriatr Oncol. 2016;7(6):479–91.
26. Lin HS, Watts JN, Peel NM, Hubbard RE. Frailty and post-operative outcomes in older surgical patients: a systematic review. BMC Geriatr. 2016;16(1):157.
27. Stoicea N, Baddigam R, Wajahn J, et al. The gap between clinical research and standard of care: a review of frailty assessment scales in perioperative surgical settings. Front Public Health. 2016;4:150.
28. Bettelli G. Preoperative evaluation in geriatric surgery: comorbidity, functional status and pharmacological history. Minerva Anestesiol. 2011;77(6):637–46.

29. Robinson TN, Wu DS, Pointer L, et al. Simple frailty score predicts postoperative complications across surgical specialties. Am J Surg. 2013;206:544–50.
30. Robinson TN, Walston JD, Brummel NE, et al. Frailty for surgeons: review of a national institute on aging conference on frailty for specialists. J Am Coll Surg. 2015;221(6):1083–92.
31. Preston SD, Southall ARD, Nel M, Das SK. Geriatric surgery is about disease, not age. J R Soc Med. 2008;101(8):409–15.
32. Jung P, Pereira MA, Hiebert B, et al. The impact of frailty on postoperative delirium in cardiac surgery patients. J Thorac Cardiovasc Surg. 2015;149(3):869–75.e1–2.
33. Revenig LM, Canter DJ, Taylor MD, et al. Too frail for surgery? Initial results of a large multidisciplinary prospective study examining preoperative variables predictive of poor surgical outcomes. J Am Coll Surg. 2013;217(4):665–70.e1.
34. Kristjansson SR, Nesbakken A, Jordhøy MS, et al. Comprehensive geriatric assessment can predict complications in elderly patients after elective surgery for colorectal cancer: a prospective observational cohort study. Crit Rev Oncol Hematol. 2010;76(3):208–17.
35. Berrut G, Andrieu S. Araujo de Carvalho I, et al. Promoting access to innovation for frail old persons. IAGG (International Association of Gerontology and Geriatrics), WHO (World Health Organization) and SFGG (Société Française de Gériatrie et de Gérontologie) Workshop –Athens January 20–21, 2012. J Nutr Health Aging. 2013;17(8):688–93.

Surgical Risk and Operative Management in Geriatric Surgery

3

Andrea Polistena, Stefano Avenia, Giuseppe Cavallaro, Giuliano D'Onghia, Monica Pellegrino, Alessandro Sanguinetti, and Nicola Avenia

3.1 Introduction

The demographic shift toward an aging population is one of the most significant healthcare challenges of the twenty-first century. Globally, improvements in public health, sanitation, and chronic disease management have contributed to a rapidly expanding elderly population. According to the United Nations, the number of individuals aged 65 and older is projected to reach nearly 1.5 billion by 2050 [1]. This will result in an unprecedented increase in demand for surgical interventions, ranging from elective orthopedic procedures to emergent abdominal and thoracic operations.

Surgery in the elderly presents a paradox: while older adults stand to benefit greatly from interventions that alleviate pain, restore function, or treat life-threatening disease, they also face heightened risks of complications and poorer recovery trajectories. The decision to operate must therefore be individualized, incorporating not only clinical risk but also patient preferences, functional status,

A. Polistena (✉) · G. D'Onghia · M. Pellegrino
Department of Surgery, Sapienza University of Rome, Policlinico Umberto I, Rome, Italy
e-mail: andrea.polistena@uniroma1.it; giuliano.donghia@uniroma1.it; monica.pellegrino@uniroma1.it

S. Avenia
Hepato-biliary and Liver Transplantation Unit, AORN Cardarelli, Naples, Italy
e-mail: stefano.avenia@aocardarelli.it

G. Cavallaro
Department of Medical-Surgical Sciences and Biotechnologies, Sapienza University of Rome-Polo Pontino, ICOT Hospital, Latina (Rome), Italy
e-mail: giuseppe.cavallaro@uniroma1.it

A. Sanguinetti · N. Avenia
Department of Surgery, Perugia University, Azienda Ospedaliera S. Maria, Terni, Italy
e-mail: a.sanguinetti@aospterni.it; nicola.avenia@unipg.it

P. Carcoforo, F. Catena (eds.), *Geriatric Surgery*, Updates in Surgery,
https://doi.org/10.1007/978-3-032-24281-5_3

and long-term goals [2–5]. This chapter explores the complex interplay between aging physiology, comorbidities, risk stratification, perioperative management, and ethical considerations in geriatric surgery, offering a comprehensive view for clinicians involved in the care of elderly surgical patients.

3.2 Epidemiology of Surgery in Older Adults

In high-income countries, nearly half of all surgical procedures are performed in patients aged 65 years and above. In the United States, Medicare data suggest that adults over 65 undergo more than 20 million surgical procedures annually. In Europe, approximately 45% of general surgical admissions involve elderly patients, with similar trends reported in Asia [3].

The types of procedures most commonly performed are:

- Elective surgery: Joint replacements, cataract extraction, colorectal resections, cholecystectomy, and coronary revascularization.
- Emergency surgery: Hip fracture repair, emergency laparotomy for bowel obstruction, perforated viscus, ruptured abdominal aortic aneurysm.

While high-resource countries report declining perioperative mortality due to improvements in anesthesia and postoperative care, low- and middle-income countries face challenges including limited access to intensive care, shortage of trained surgeons, and inadequate postoperative support systems. Elderly patients in these regions often present late with advanced disease, compounding surgical risk [3].

3.3 Physiological Changes with Aging

Aging is associated with progressive decline in the physiological reserve of multiple organ systems (Table 3.1). This reduced homeostatic capacity results in increased vulnerability to surgical stressors such as anesthesia, bleeding, hypoxia, and sepsis [2–5]. The combination of multiple organs' progressive decline in physiological

Table 3.1 Summary of age-related physiological changes and implications

System	Change	Implication
Cardiovascular	↑ Arterial stiffness, ↓ Compliance	Ischemia, BP lability
Pulmonary	↓ Vital capacity, ↓ Recoil	Atelectasis, pneumonia risk
Renal	↓ GFR, ↓ Perfusion	Drug toxicity, AKI
Hepatic	↓ Enzyme activity	Altered metabolism
CNS	↓ Neuroplasticity	Delirium, cognitive decline
Musculoskeletal	Sarcopenia, osteoporosis	Frailty, falls
Immune	↓ T-cell function	Poor infection response

AKI acute kidney failure, *BP* blood pressure, *CNS* central nervous system, *GFR* glomerular filtration rate reserve contributes to define frailty as a medical syndrome with multiple causes and contributors, a syndrome characterized by diminished strength and endurance, and reduced physiological function, with a reduced ability to adapt to environmental changes which might be particularly relevant in surgical patients regarding their compliance with surgical treatments. Therefore, perioperative identification of high-risk groups for postoperative frailty is crucial for optimizing clinical decision-making [4–7].

Physical frailty differs from multimorbidity. Both are common, but multimorbidity is more pervasive, being present in 3 in 4 individuals older than 65 years and 1 in 4 of those younger than 65 [8]. However, some patients experience persistent postoperative frailty, leading to delayed recovery and suboptimal surgical outcomes. This substantially diminishes the clinical benefits even of elective surgery for these patients [8].

3.4 Risk Stratification in Geriatric Surgery and Tools for Evaluation

Risk assessment is critical in surgical decision-making for elderly patients. Traditional tools are insufficient when used alone, and comprehensive assessments that include frailty, comorbidities, and psychosocial context are necessary.

The most commonly used tools are [9] (Table 3.2):

- American Society of Anesthesiologists (ASA) Physical Status Classification: simple and widely used but limited in predictive accuracy.
- Charlson Comorbidity Index (CCI): predicts 10-year mortality based on comorbidities.
- Frailty indices: Fried Frailty Index, Clinical Frailty Scale, and Edmonton Frail Scale.
- Vulnerable Elders Surgical Pathways and Outcomes Assessment (VESPA): combines age, comorbidities, functional and cognitive status.

Table 3.2 Comparison of strengths and limitations of risk stratification tools

Tool	Focus	Strengths	Limitations
ASA	General fitness	Simple, widely used	Subjective, poor granularity
Charlson Index	Comorbidities	Predicts long-term survival	Not procedure-specific
Frailty Indices	Functional reserve	Strong predictor of complications	Takes time
VESPA	Holistic	Combines multiple domains	Less widely validated
ACS-NSQIP	Perioperative risk	Individualized risk	Requires database input

ACS-NSQIP American College of Surgeons—National Surgical Quality Improvement Program, *ASA* American Society of Anesthesiologists, *VESPA* Vulnerable Elders Surgical Pathways and Outcomes Assessment

- American College of Surgeons—National Surgical Quality Improvement Program (ACS-NSQIP) Risk Calculator: provides individualized risk estimates for morbidity and mortality.

3.5 Preoperative Evaluation and Optimization

Preoperative optimization is essential for reducing surgical complications in elderly patients. Physicians need to identify the older population at a high risk of persistent postoperative frailty after elective surgery. Therefore, preventive measures can be implemented in advance to reduce the risk of postoperative complications, such as improving nutritional status, managing chronic diseases, improving cardiac and respiratory functions. This not only benefits the patient but also reduces the increase in total hospitalization costs in elective surgical procedures [2, 9].

The key areas of focus are:

- Comorbidities: Optimize management of hypertension, coronary artery disease, chronic kidney disease, and chronic obstructive pulmonary disease [10, 11].
- Nutrition: Screen for malnutrition using tools such as the Mini Nutritional Assessment (MNA). Nutritional prehabilitation with protein-rich supplements improves outcomes [12].
- Polypharmacy: Review medications to minimize drug interactions and inappropriate prescriptions. High-risk medications (anticholinergics, benzodiazepines, anticoagulants) require special attention [13].
- Cognition and function: Screen for dementia, depression, and frailty. Functional assessments providing predictive value for postoperative recovery [14, 15].
- Prehabilitation: A multimodal program including exercise, nutrition, and psychological support has been shown to reduce postoperative complications [16].

3.6 Perioperative Management

The perioperative management includes several steps counting anesthetic and therapeutic considerations and delirium prevention strategies.

Anesthetic considerations [14–17]:

- Age-related changes in pharmacokinetics demand careful dosing.
- Regional anesthesia may reduce postoperative delirium risk.
- Multimodal anesthesia protocols are preferred to minimize opioid exposure.

Therapeutic considerations [12, 18, 19]:

- Fluid management: Use of goal-directed therapy avoids volume overload and renal hypoperfusion.

Table 3.3 Delirium prevention strategies

Strategy	Rationale
Avoid benzodiazepines	Reduce deliriogenic effects
Maintain orientation	Decrease confusion
Early mobilization	Improve function, reduce delirium
Hydration	Prevent metabolic imbalances
Glasses/hearing aids	Reduce sensory deprivation

- Temperature control: Older adults are prone to hypothermia, increasing bleeding and infection risk.
- Monitoring: Continuous hemodynamic monitoring is essential, especially in frail patients.

Delirium prevention strategies [14, 15] (Table 3.3):

- Avoid benzodiazepines and deliriogenic drugs.
- Maintain orientation (clocks, calendars, familiar objects).
- Encourage early mobilization and adequate hydration.
- Ensure appropriate sensory aids (glasses, hearing aids).

3.7 Specialty-Specific Implications in the Pre- and Perioperative Evaluation

3.7.1 General Surgery

Regarding major abdominal surgery, elderly patients have increased rates of postoperative morbidity and mortality and a later stage of disease, and are more likely to have emergency surgery [20]. Minor complications, mainly respiratory complications occur more frequently in the elderly. Preoperative lung capacity tests might aid in identifying elders at risk. Major complications consist mainly of surgical technical complications such as postoperative bleeding, anastomotic leak, intra-abdominal abscesses, and abdominal wall dehiscence, indicating that standardized surgical techniques ensure similar rates for major complications regardless of age, nevertheless suggesting an accurate patient selection for major abdominal procedures [20]. Guidelines recommend for elderly elective oncologic patients the use of a multidimensional geriatric assessment scale before embarking on active medical oncology treatment and before undergoing major surgery [21]. General surgery operations in the emergency setting are associated with a nearly two-fold and five-fold increase of risks. Accurate preoperative identification of frailty is crucial for risk stratification and informed decision-making ensuring that patients receive tailored treatments based on their ability to withstand operative stressors. Selection of the appropriate frailty instrument is fundamental in this setting and a standardized guideline on the use of these instruments is strongly recommended [22].

3.7.2 Orthopedics

Aging and frailty are highly correlated with sarcopenia, bone density and nutritional status. Grip strength and gait speed tests have certain advantages in reflecting muscle reserves and physiological status and are widely used in the assessment of frailty in older adults [23–26]. This is because these tests cannot reflect the true and objective physiological reserves of these patients. Poor preoperative grip strength and gait speed often indicate a lower physiological reserve capacity, higher sensitivity to adverse events, and an increased likelihood of surgery triggering or exacerbating frailty. Postoperative activity reduction, resulting in functional decline and muscle atrophy, may further contribute to a vicious cycle of frailty [27]. Osteoporosis, a common metabolic bone condition primarily affecting geriatrics globally, weakens bones and raises fracture risk. Prior osteoporotic fractures heighten susceptibility to further fractures, notably hip fractures, impacting outcomes post-surgical management [28]. This emphasizes the need for meticulous preoperative preparation, proactive osteoporosis treatment, and prudent rehabilitation [29–31].

3.7.3 Cardiac Surgery

Despite surgical innovations and advancements in surgical technology, the decision on whether to proceed with invasive interventions in this patient population remains a challenge owing to an increased risk of perioperative-related complications. Cardiac surgery is an invasive treatment, and frail patients may benefit more from less invasive percutaneous procedures for coronary or valvular disease, such as percutaneous coronary intervention (PCI), transcatheter aortic valve implantation (TAVI), and transcatheter edge-to-edge mitral valve repair. Patients whose goals prioritize comfort and functional status may select less invasive procedures or optimal medical therapy if an intervention's risks outweigh its potential benefit. For those patients undergoing cardiac surgery, postoperative early rehabilitation, both in-hospital and in the immediate post-discharge period, helps to reduce the adverse effects of prolonged bed rest and decrease the risk of postoperative complications, by enhancing autonomic cardiac function at discharge, and shortening the length of hospital stay. Furthermore, occupational therapy may also improve timely, appropriate, and safe discharges of frail patients guaranteeing compliance with the patient's engagement in daily tasks and enhancing the patient's overall quality of life [31]. Preinterventional frailty assessments for patients scheduled for cardiac surgery were recently published [32–34]. After a complete evaluation of the patient's risk, there is noteworthy evidence that in various areas (aerobic conditioning, diabetic control, respiratory muscle training, lifestyle modification, psychoeducation, and sleep), intervening prior to cardiac surgery can improve outcomes [31]. At present, the Pre-operative Rehabilitation for Reduction of Hospitalization After Coronary Bypass and Valvular Surgery (PREHAB) study is an ongoing multicenter randomized controlled trial aiming to examine the effect of prehabilitation, in which frail patients awaiting cardiac surgery either receive the current standard of care or participate in an 8-week exercise/education program at a community-based cardiac rehabilitation center [35, 36].

3.7.4 Neurosurgery

In recent decades neurosurgery presented a rapid technical and technological evolution leading to improved outcomes and larger inclusion of surgical candidates. In elderly patients, according to large experiences reported in the literature, the causes of hospital admission for neurosurgical disorders include: occlusive cerebrovascular disease (40%), spinal degenerative myeloradiculopathy (14%), tumors (7%), trauma (5.4%), and intracranial hematomas (4%). In the older patients, aged 85 and over, occlusive cerebrovascular disease is the leading pathology, followed by subdural hematomas, spinal degenerative myeloradiculopathy, trigeminal neuralgias, hydrocephalus, vascular anomalies, and tumors. In the past, older age was believed to be a contraindication for surgery; however, the increased life expectancy, number, and health of this population suggest a larger inclusion of potential elderly surgical candidates, based on an optimized preoperative evaluation and clear identification of patients at higher risk [37]. In an elderly patient population with brain metastases requiring surgery, the presence of multiple lesions, infratentorial location and frail condition were shown as independent predictors of worse overall survival [38]. Elective spinal surgery can be safely performed even in well-selected patients over 80 years of age. However, the extent of surgery and low performance status scores are associated with increased complications from spinal surgery in octogenarians [39]. The frailer patients with glioblastoma are less likely to undergo surgical resection, have a longer hospital stay, experience more complications, and have shorter overall survival. Furthermore, frailty was associated with outcomes independent of age, functional status, cardiovascular risk, and comorbidity [40].

3.8 The Role of the Multidisciplinary Team

Although clinical practice guidelines and publications recommend preoperative multidisciplinary team (MDT) meetings as standard practice in the perioperative care of high-risk surgical patients, in many hospitals such meetings have yet to become routine in all surgical fields, having been instead mostly standardized in specific fields only. Implementing a preoperative MDT meeting to optimize patient care before surgery improves outcomes and facilitates shared decision-making, particularly for high-risk patients. Currently, no guidance exists to identify high-risk patients for whom preoperative MDT discussion may be useful. Most studies describing preoperative MDT discussions for high-risk patients use clinical judgment regarding the harm-benefit ratio of the intended surgery as the main method to identify high-risk patients. Initial patient selection for an MDT discussion, mostly by the anesthesiologist, must be considered to improve optimal care and contain patients' surgical risk [41].

3.9 Operative Strategies

Operative decision-making must consider both the technical aspects of surgery and the patient's overall condition.

Specialty-specific implications must be considered:

- General surgery: Minimally invasive techniques (laparoscopy) reduce wound complications but require careful patient selection due to pneumoperitoneum effects. Application of robotic surgery offers minimally invasive benefits, but longer operative times and greater resource use. Percutaneous treatments are recommended in high-risk patients whenever possible and non-operative treatment applied to those patients not fit for surgery [20–22].
- Orthopedics: Hip fracture repair is often lifesaving; early surgery (<48 hours) reduces mortality and complications [23–25, 29].
- Cardiac surgery: Transcatheter or endovascular approaches (transcatheter aortic valve replacement [TAVR], endovascular aortic aneurysm repair [EVAR]) are increasingly favored over open surgery in elderly high-risk patients, with similar considerations for vascular surgery [32–34].
- Neurosurgery: Craniotomy for subdural hematoma and cerebral tumors may restore function and increase oncological prognosis but carries high perioperative risk in frail patients [37–39].

3.10 Postoperative Care

Elderly patients face unique postoperative challenges.

Enhanced Recovery After Surgery (ERAS®) in geriatrics [12, 18, 19]:

- Early oral feeding reduces infection and length of stay.
- Multimodal analgesia minimizes opioid-related side effects.
- Early mobilization on postoperative day 1 prevents functional decline.

Complication prevention:

- Delirium: Prevent with orientation, minimize restraints, ensure sleep hygiene [14, 15].
- Infection: Strict asepsis, early removal of catheters and drains [18, 19].
- Venous thromboembolism: Pharmacologic prophylaxis combined with mechanical compression and early mobilization [18, 19].
- Pressure ulcers: Frequent repositioning and specialized mattresses.

Rehabilitation [42]:

- Early physiotherapy and occupational therapy restore independence.

- Transition to skilled nursing facilities or home health programs should be planned before discharge.

3.11 Future Directions

Emerging trends in geriatric surgery include precision medicine (genomic and biomarker-based risk stratification), application of artificial intelligence (machine learning models using electronic health records to predict surgical outcomes), telemedicine (improved follow-up and early complication detection in older adults with mobility limitations), implementation of geriatric surgical programs with institution of dedicated multidisciplinary boards (geriatricians, surgeons, anesthesiologists, physiotherapists) to improve care coordination and outcomes, increased focus on ethical issues and patient preference.

3.12 Conclusion

The management of elderly surgical patients demands a multidisciplinary and individualized approach. Surgeons must integrate risk stratification tools, optimization strategies, and ethical frameworks to ensure surgery provides not only longer life but also better quality of life. As the aging population grows, geriatric surgery will remain at the forefront of surgical innovation.

References

1. Etzioni DA, Liu JH, Maggard MA, Ko CY. The aging population and its impact on the surgery workforce. Ann Surg. 2003;238(2):170–7.
2. Chow WB, Rosenthal RA, Merkow RP, et al. Optimal preoperative assessment of the geriatric surgical patient: a best practices guideline from the American College of Surgeons National Surgical Quality Improvement Program and the American Geriatrics Society. J Am Coll Surg. 2012;215(4):453–66.
3. Partridge JS, Harari D, Dhesi JK. Frailty in the older surgical patient: a review. Age Ageing. 2012;41(2):142–7.
4. Makary MA, Segev DL, Pronovost PJ, et al. Frailty as a predictor of surgical outcomes in older patients. J Am Coll Surg. 2010;210(6):901–8.
5. Hamel MB, Henderson WG, Khuri SF, Daley J. Surgical outcomes for patients aged 80 and older: morbidity and mortality from major noncardiac surgery. J Am Geriatr Soc. 2005;53(3):424–9.
6. Dai BZ, Zhou LL, Mei YJ. Old age security in rural China: there is a long way to go. Chin Med J. 2013;126(22):4348–53.
7. Davinelli S, Corbi G, Scapagnini G. Frailty syndrome: a target for functional nutrients? Mech Ageing Dev. 2021;195:111441.
8. Tinetti ME, Fried TR, Boyd CM. Designing health care for the most common chronic condition - multimorbidity. JAMA. 2012;307(23):2493–4.
9. Rockwood K, Song X, MacKnight C, et al. A global clinical measure of fitness and frailty in elderly people. CMAJ. 2005;173(5):489–95.

10. Oresanya LB, Lyons WL, Finlayson E. Preoperative assessment of the older patient: a narrative review. JAMA. 2014;311(20):2110–20.
11. Mohanty S, Rosenthal RA, Russell MM, et al. Optimal perioperative management of the geriatric patient: a best practices guideline from the American College of Surgeons NSQIP and the American Geriatrics Society. J Am Coll Surg. 2016;222(5):930–47.
12. Molenaar CJL, Minnella EM, Coca-Martinez M, et al. Effect of multimodal prehabilitation on reducing postoperative complications and enhancing functional capacity following colorectal cancer surgery: the PREHAB randomized clinical trial. JAMA Surg. 2023;158(6):572–81.
13. Wang Z, Liu T, Su Q, et al. Prevalence of polypharmacy in elderly population worldwide: a systematic review and meta-analysis. Pharmacoepidemiol Drug Saf. 2024;33(8):e5880.
14. Deiner S, Silverstein JH. Postoperative delirium and cognitive dysfunction. Br J Anaesth. 2009;103(Suppl 1):i41–6.
15. Inouye SK, Westendorp RG, Saczynski JS. Delirium in elderly people. Lancet. 2014;383(9920):911–22.
16. Kaye AD, Baluch A, Scott JT. Pain management in the elderly population: a review. Ochsner J. 2010;10(3):179–87.
17. Guay J, Parker MJ, Griffiths R, Kopp S. Peripheral nerve blocks for hip fractures. Cochrane Database Syst Rev. 2017;5(5):CD001159.
18. Kehlet H, Wilmore DW. Fast-track surgery. Br J Surg. 2005;92(1):3–4.
19. Scott MJ, Baldini G, Fearon KC, et al. Enhanced Recovery After Surgery (ERAS) for gastrointestinal surgery, part 1: pathophysiological considerations. Acta Anaesthesiol Scand. 2015;59(10):1212–31.
20. Straatman J, Van der Wielen N, Cuesta MA, et al. Major abdominal surgery in octogenarians: should high age affect surgical decision-making? Am J Surg. 2016;212(5):889–95.
21. Finlayson EV, Birkmeyer JD. Operative mortality with elective surgery in older adults. Eff Clin Pract. 2001;4(4):172–7.
22. Lavanchy JL, Holzgang MM, Haltmeier T, et al. Outcomes of emergency abdominal surgery in octogenarians: a single-center analysis. Am J Surg. 2019;218(2):248–54.
23. Soltani A, Abolhassani N, Marques-Vidal P, et al. Real-world gait speed estimation, frailty and handgrip strength: a cohort-based study. Sci Rep. 2021;11(1):18966.
24. Custodero C, Agosti P, Anton SD, et al. Effect of physical activity intervention on gait speed by frailty condition: a randomized clinical trial. J Am Med Dir Assoc. 2023;24(4):489–96.
25. Gao G, Zheng Z, Ye Z, et al. A prediction model for persistent postoperative frailty in older patients undergoing elective orthopedic surgery. Medicine (Baltimore). 2025;104(31):e43500.
26. Clegg A, Young J, Iliffe S, et al. Frailty in elderly people. Lancet. 2013;381(9868):752–62.
27. Courtney-Brooks M, Tellawi AR, Scalici J, et al. Frailty: an outcome predictor for elderly gynecologic oncology patients. Gynecol Oncol. 2012;126(1):20–4.
28. Nichols CI, Vose JG. Patient comorbidity status and incremental total hospitalization costs in elective orthopedic procedures. Orthopedics. 2016;39(4):237–46.
29. Dawod MS, Alswerki MN, Yasin MS, et al. Impact of prior fragility fracture on patient's mortality, outcomes, and complications after hip fracture surgery. BMC Musculoskelet Disord. 2025;26(1):593.
30. Padegimas EM, Osei DA. Evaluation and treatment of osteoporotic distal radius fracture in the elderly patient. Curr Rev Musculoskelet Med. 2013;6(1):41–6.
31. Afilalo J, Lauck S, Kim DH, et al. Frailty in older adults undergoing aortic valve replacement: the FRAILTY-AVR study. J Am Coll Cardiol. 2017;70(6):689–700.
32. Chandiramani A, Ali JM. Frailty in cardiac surgery - assessment tools, impact on outcomes, and optimisation strategies: a narrative review. J Cardiovasc Dev Dis. 2025;12(4):127.
33. Niebauer J, Bäck C, Bischoff-Ferrari HA, et al. Preinterventional frailty assessment in patients scheduled for cardiac surgery or transcatheter aortic valve implantation: a consensus statement of the European Association for Cardio-Thoracic Surgery (EACTS) and the European Association of Preventive Cardiology (EAPC) of the European Society of Cardiology (ESC). Eur J Prev Cardiol. 2024;31(2):146–81.

34. Nguyenhuy M, Chang J, Xu R, et al. The Fried frailty phenotype in patients undergoing cardiac surgery: a systematic review and meta-analysis. Heart Surg Forum. 2022;25(5):E652–9.
35. Western MJ, Malkowski OS. Associations of the Short Physical Performance Battery (SPPB) with adverse health outcomes in older adults: a 14-year follow-up from the English longitudinal study of ageing (ELSA). Int J Environ Res Public Health. 2022;19(23):16319.
36. Stammers AN, Kehler DS, Afilalo J, et al. Protocol for the PREHAB study - pre-operative rehabilitation for reduction of hospitalization after coronary bypass and valvular surgery: a randomised controlled trial. BMJ Open. 2015;5(3):e007250.
37. Dujovny M, Charbel F, Berman SK, et al. Geriatric neurosurgery. Surg Neurol. 1987;28(1):10–6.
38. Heimann M, Schäfer N, Bode C, et al. Outcome of elderly patients with surgically treated brain metastases. Front Oncol. 2021;11:713965.
39. Mihailidis HG, Manners S, Churilov L, Quan GMY. Is spinal surgery safe in octogenarians? ANZ J Surg. 2017;87(7–8):605–9.
40. Cloney M, D'Amico R, Lebovic J, et al. Frailty in geriatric glioblastoma patients: a predictor of operative morbidity and outcome. World Neurosurg. 2016;89:362–7.
41. Vernooij JEM, Hobrink E, Boerlage RM, et al. Characteristics and outcome of preoperative multidisciplinary team discussions for high-risk noncardiac surgical patients in The Netherlands: a multicentre prospective observational study. Br J Anaesth. 2025;135(2):449–58.
42. Lin HS, Watts JN, Peel NM, Hubbard RE. Frailty and post-operative outcomes in older surgical patients: a systematic review. BMC Geriatr. 2016;16(1):157.

Informed Consensus and Futility

4

Bruno Amato, Rita Compagna, Mario Bellisi, Michele De Capua, Ermenegildo Furino, Ignazio Verde, Francesco Riccitelli, Salvatore Silvano, Giulia Amato, Giuseppe Vacchiano, and Domenico Tafuri

4.1 Introduction

Medical and surgical practice, being potentially capable of profoundly affecting a person's psycho-physical integrity and efficiency, and sometimes even endangering life itself, is permitted under the Italian legal system insofar as it is aimed at safeguarding health. It necessarily presupposes the patient's fundamental consent: the physician's activity, in fact, finds its precise and insurmountable limit in the patient's will, provided the latter is capable of self-determination and of freely safeguarding essential personal values such as freedom, dignity, life, health, and psycho-physical integrity.

B. Amato (✉)
Department of Public Health, University of Naples Federico II, Policlinico Federico II, Naples, Italy
e-mail: bruno.amato@unina.it

R. Compagna
Vascular Surgery, AORN Cardarelli, Naples, Italy
e-mail: rita.compagna@gmail.com

M. Bellisi
P. Giaccone Teaching Hospital, University of Palermo, Palermo, Italy
e-mail: mariobellisi@libero.it

M. De Capua
Spedali Civili, Brescia, Italy
e-mail: michele.decapua90@gmail.com

E. Furino
Department of Emergency Surgery, Umberto I Medical School, Sapienza University of Rome, Rome, Italy
e-mail: er.furino@gmail.com

I. Verde
University of Campania Luigi Vanvitelli, Medical School, Naples, Italy
e-mail: dottignazioverde@gmail.com

P. Carcoforo, F. Catena (eds.), *Geriatric Surgery*, Updates in Surgery,
https://doi.org/10.1007/978-3-032-24281-5_4

Consent to medical treatment therefore represents—except in specific cases such as compulsory health treatments or situations of danger to the patient's life—the most effective means available to the patient to safeguard and defend their values and rights. Any medical act performed without due consent constitutes a serious ethical and legal breach, inevitably subject to severe censure.

This perspective, which recognizes the patient as a person and draws direct inspiration from the Italian Constitution [1], is clearly enshrined in the Code of Medical Ethics [2]. It has been acknowledged by case law since 1990 [3], reaffirmed in numerous subsequent rulings [4], and fully consecrated through the enactment of a specific law [5]. Consequently, no medical treatment may be initiated or continued, except in particular circumstances, without the free and informed consent of the person concerned. This promotes and strengthens the relationship of care and trust between physician and patient.

4.2 The Central Role of Information

Patient consent to a medical act must always be preceded by adequate information, which cannot be relegated to a mere prerequisite but assumes a fundamental role in its acquisition. The duty to provide information constitutes an autonomous and specific obligation of protection toward the patient, in fulfillment of their primary right to know the clinical data that concern them, of which the physician is merely a qualified interpreter.

Information regarding the patient's condition, diagnostic-therapeutic pathway, possible risks, alternatives, and potential complications is therefore the key element enabling the patient's full self-determination [5]. Information must be clear, comprehensive, adapted to the patient's mental and social condition, and delivered calmly—avoiding both an excessively negative portrayal of reality and the exclusion of possible positive outcomes, even in cases of poor prognosis.

F. Riccitelli
Sanatorio Triestino Clinic, Trieste, Italy
e-mail: riccitellifrancesco@gmail.com

S. Silvano
Department of Public Health, ASL Novara, Novara, Italy
e-mail: salv.silvano@gmail.com

G. Amato · D. Tafuri
Department of Medical, Motor and Wellness Sciences, Parthenope University, Naples, Italy
e-mail: giu_amat@hotmail.it; domenico.tafuri@uniparthenope.it

G. Vacchiano
Department of Law, Economics, Management and Quantitative Methods (DEMM), University of Sannio, Benevento, Italy
e-mail: vacchiano952@gmail.com

A correct approach to information must be patient-centered and tailored to the individual's actual capacities so as to be fully comprehensible. Comprehensibility is indispensable for valid consent, and it must be structured according to both the intrinsic characteristics of the patient (socio-cultural level, attentional capacity, psychological experience of illness) and the quality and quantity of the information provided.

To facilitate this, the Italian Society of Surgery has developed information templates for common surgical procedures, to be presented before any intervention and during preliminary assessments. However, the uncritical delivery of a mere pre-printed form, especially immediately before surgery, does not relieve the surgeon of responsibility [6]. Information must be read, explained, discussed, and understood. The form thus represents an additional tool, not a substitute for the physician's duty to inform.

Ultimately, information must be conceived as an osmotic process between physician and patient, with questions, clarifications, and dialogue, culminating in a "shared decision" [7]. For minimally invasive and non-dangerous procedures a simple explanation of the examination method and the quick acquisition of consent—even verbal and sometimes implicit—is sufficient. Relatively dangerous activities, with potential risk to the patient's life or health, must be performed, but the information provided and the consent obtained must be documented in written form and will become an integral part of the clinical records, attesting to the proper and justifiable medical approach.

4.3 The Nature of Consent

Consent does not require particular formulas but must always be personal, free, informed, expressed by a competent individual, and revocable. Specifically:

- It must come personally from the patient, except where legal representation applies.
- It must be expressed by a patient capable of understanding and decision-making at the time consent is given.
- It must be freely formed, not the result of coercion, deception, or misrepresentation.
- It must be contemporaneous with the treatment itself.
- It is revocable, at least until it is technically possible to interrupt treatment.
- It should generally be obtained by the physician performing the treatment, although in healthcare facilities it may also be obtained by another member of the team.
- It must correspond to each distinct phase of care (diagnostic tests, anesthesia, surgery).
- It cannot be *ad personam* in the public setting, meaning it cannot be conditioned upon the intervention being performed by a specific physician.

4.4 Consent, Refusal, and the Elderly Patient

Elderly patients with reduced cognitive or intellectual capacity often lack legal representatives or advance directives. In such cases, the surgeon's relational role must be especially attentive, fostering dialogue and understanding to allow even limited self-determination.

In this regard, a useful operational approach has been proposed, based on the observance of three specific, fundamental stages of dialogue between the physician and the patient: choice, option, and decision [8]. Thus, once the problem has been identified and the diagnosis established, the patient may be presented with possible diagnostic/therapeutic choices; subsequently, the various operative options will be examined in detail, together with their potential difficulties and expected outcomes; finally, the patient will decide which diagnostic/therapeutic option to pursue. It should nonetheless always be emphasized that the patient must be supported in making their choice of intervention, in order to reach a "shared decision" [9].

Sometimes, conflicts could arise between the patient's (or family's) requesting for an aggressive intervention and the physician's assessment of its futility. Such disagreements may be referred to the Guardianship Judge, who may authorize either treatment or abstention.

Furthermore, advance healthcare directives may be taken into account, where present, which provide that every person capable of self-determination may, in anticipation of a possible, future incapacity, express their will, their consent, or their refusal with regard to healthcare treatments or interventions to which they might be subjected [5]. It should also be noted that the treating physician, together with the patient, may draft a care plan which, by anticipating the progression of the disease and the possibility of a future surgical intervention, may justify the procedure or its omission in the event of the patient's subsequent incapacity [5]. However, such directives are devoid of effect when they are manifestly incongruent with the specific condition of the patient, or they may be legitimately superseded by the availability of therapies not known to the patient at the time of the drafting of such directives.

Moreover, when there is a divergence regarding necessary treatment between the physician and the patient, or their legal representative, the possibility arises of appealing to the Guardianship Judge, who may, by means of their ruling, legitimize the proposed intervention.

Nonetheless, beyond judicial involvement, communication remains essential to explain the utility or the lack of utility of interventions.

Such a possibility, though indeed uncommon, presupposes a surgical procedure that can be planned; however, should there be the need for urgent intervention, the surgeon, due to their specific position of responsibility towards the patient, is authorized to act—particularly when the intervention is easy to perform and characterized by a favorable risk/benefit ratio. Nevertheless, elderly patients with reduced cognitive and intellectual capacity do not always have the support of their legal representative, nor are advance healthcare directives or shared care plans always in place [10].

In such cases, the physician's relational approach must necessarily be particularly attentive, thoughtful, and proportionate, so as to allow even these individuals to exercise their, albeit limited, capacity for self-determination. Indeed, the patient's request for help, their particular condition of suffering, as well as the recognized authority of the surgeon to dictate the timing and manner of the diagnostic/therapeutic intervention, condition a relationship increasingly unbalanced in favor of the professional, who is called upon, through intelligent listening, dialogue, and understanding, to render the doctor–patient relationship increasingly symmetrical and equal. In this relationship, the two actors are: one, free to propose a given intervention to address a specific diagnostic/therapeutic need; the other, free to accept it, postpone it, or refuse it based on their own particular needs, convictions, or circumstances. However, the patient must be supported in reaching a decision.

This particularly delicate and complex approach is, in fact, quite problematic, and the literature suggests overcoming the rational apathy of a patient whose indifference to treatment hinders their care [11], while at the same time highlighting the difficult choices to be made, especially with respect to high-risk surgical procedures with potentially unfavorable outcomes [12].

Yet, the search for a therapy to which the patient—and especially their family members—turn in the hope of achieving an improved clinical condition, perhaps through a dangerously destructive surgical intervention, highly disabling and with uncertain outcomes, and the proposal suggested and explained by the physician, aware of the futility of such a procedure, sometimes generates a profound, insurmountable conflict of opinions. In such circumstances, the surgeon is called upon to make a particularly delicate and complex assessment, both on the technical/operative level and on the ethical level, which does not always coincide with the will of the patient. Indeed, the patient's concrete and objective conditions must be duly considered, since they do not always permit compliance with their request: either because of their specific clinical condition, which does not allow them to positively withstand surgical and anesthetic stress; or due to the peculiar nature of the disease affecting them; or, finally, because of foreseeable outcomes not always characterized by a favorable cost/benefit ratio. In this regard, it is essential to emphasize the physician's freedom of decision: they are not obliged to perform procedures contrary to their technical assessments, their ethical/deontological convictions, or the rules of good clinical practice. Likewise, the patient cannot demand a treatment that contravenes medical standards and technical indications.

4.5 Medical Futility and Abstentionism

In such cases, a particular communicative ability is required, in order to make the patient understand the lack of usefulness of the requested and expected intervention [13], and to avoid performing a procedure devoid of effectiveness, thereby constituting an instance of medical futility [14].

To justify the physician's technical/operative abstention and to deem an intervention futile, the "quantitative" aspects of the requested treatment have been considered, such as the success rates of the last 100 similar procedures [15], or the possibility that the intervention may only improve certain functions of the patient without altering their disease or dependence on intensive medical care [16]. Furthermore, emphasis has been placed on the absence of a reasonable probability of improving the patient's quality of life, and on the need to employ significant resources without a reasonable hope of achieving any concrete improvement in the patient's living conditions [17].

Recently, the use of artificial intelligence (AI) in defining the futility of urgent surgical interventions has also been proposed and emphasized [18]. Indeed, the application of AI in medicine, through the analysis of an innumerable series of data examined rapidly and accurately, constitutes a valuable aid in the diagnostic/therapeutic process and could offer undeniable support in the delicate decisions that both the patient and the surgeon are called upon to make—particularly in assessing the morbidity and mortality associated with a given surgical procedure—by complementing existing decision-making models [19–21]. However, while the intervention of AI in medical practice may provide numerous operational advantages [22], this tool cannot be applied mechanically and indiscriminately, but must be carefully considered and evaluated [23].

The issue in question is extremely complex and delicate, and presupposes an in-depth evaluation of the case by the physician. It unfortunately risks being entirely subjective, shaped by specific personal beliefs, influenced by social, cultural, and religious factors that are difficult to assess, by the fear of possible repercussions, and always characterized by an unavoidable degree of uncertainty. Such a decision, however, can only be made in the "best interest of the patient," who, whenever possible, must necessarily be involved in the decision-making process, with the physician explaining the difficulties, the uncertain outcomes, the lack of unequivocal indications for surgery, and the reasons discouraging its performance. Indeed, although medical practice is fundamentally experimental and always in search of new solutions to improve the patient's lifespan and quality of life, it must be acknowledged that technical/operative abstention may be justifiable in certain circumstances—when it is based on objectively verifiable criteria and data, supported by sound scientific arguments, and free from unilateral assessments typical of a paternalistic medical model, now outdated. At the same time, the patient's will must always, where possible, be sought and respected, since old age, operational difficulties and limited economic resources must never go so far as to deny access to potential innovative technical solutions aimed at safeguarding the patient's fundamental right to health.

4.6 Conclusion

Balancing technical and ethical requirements defines the very essence of the medical profession. Medicine cannot be reduced to a bureaucratic application of techniques or guidelines but must always adapt to the unique circumstances of each case, particularly in geriatric patients. Above all, interventions must be tailored to the real needs of the ill person who, especially in conditions of fragility, must always be respected, adequately assisted, and never abandoned.

References

1. Art. 32 Italian Constitution: "No one may be obliged to undergo any given medical treatment except as provided by the law. Under no circumstances may the law violate the limits imposed by respect for the human person".
2. Art. 35 Code of Medical Ethics – Informed consent and dissent: "The physician shall not initiate nor continue diagnostic procedures and/or therapeutic interventions without first obtaining informed consent, or in the presence of informed dissent".
3. Court of Assizes of Florence, Judgment of 18 October 1990.
4. Court of Milan, Judgment no. 2331 of 25.02.2005; Supreme Court of Cassation, Civil Division III, Judgment no. 2239 of 19.10.2006; Supreme Court of Cassation, Criminal Division IV, Judgment no. 37077 of 30.09.2008; Supreme Court of Cassation, Civil Division III, Judgment no. 20806 of 29.09.2009; Supreme Court of Cassation, Criminal Division IV, Judgment no. 48322 of 17.12.2009; Supreme Court of Cassation, Civil Division III, Judgment no. 2847 of 09.02.2010; Supreme Court of Cassation, Civil Division III, Judgment no. 3075 of 11.02.2010; Supreme Court of Cassation, Civil Division III, Judgment no. 19220 of 20.08.2013; Supreme Court of Cassation, Civil Division III, Judgment no. 27751 of 11.12.2013; Supreme Court of Cassation, Criminal Division IV, Judgment no. 2347 of 20.01.2014.
5. Italian Law no. 219 of 22.12.2017 – Provisions on informed consent and advance healthcare directives.
6. Cocanour CS. Informed consent – it's more than a signature on a piece of paper. Am J Surg. 2017;214(6):993–7.
7. Grady C. Enduring and emerging challenges of informed consent. N Engl J Med. 2015;372(9):885–62.
8. Elwyn G, Frosch D, Thomson R, et al. Shared decision making: a model for clinical practice. J Gen Intern Med. 2012;27(10):1361–7.
9. Entwistle VA, Carter SM, Cribb A, McCaffery K. Supporting patient autonomy: the importance of clinician-patient relationships. J Gen Intern Med. 2010;25(7):741–5.
10. Giampieri M. Communication and informed consent in elderly people. Minerva Anestesiol. 2012;78(2):236–42.
11. Noah BA, Reich-Graefe R. Rational patient apathy. Seton Hall Law Rev. 2019;49(3):535–628.
12. Angelos P, Taylor LJ, Roggin K, et al. Decision-making in surgery. Ann Thorac Surg. 2024;117(6):1087–94.
13. Hickman S, Gangemi A. Going beyond "bad news": a surgical case report and systematic review of the literature surrounding futile care. Int J Surg Case Rep. 2019;59:35–40.
14. Grant SB, Modi PK, Singer EA. Futility and the care of surgical patients: ethical dilemmas. World J Surg. 2014;38(7):1631–7.
15. Schneiderman LJ. Defining medical futility and improving medical care. J Bioeth Inq. 2011;8(2):123–31.
16. Gabbay E, Calvo-Broce J, Meyer KB, et al. The empirical basis for determinations of medical futility. J Gen Intern Med. 2010;25(10):1083–9.
17. Aghabarary M, Dehghan Nayeri N. Medical futility and its challenges: a review study. J Med Ethics Hist Med. 2016;9:11.
18. Bianchi V, Misuriello F, Piras E, et al. Ethical considerations on the role of artificial intelligence in defining the futility in emergency surgery. Int J Surg. 2025;111(5):3178–84.
19. El Hechi MW, Maurer LR, Levine J, et al. Validation of the artificial intelligence-based predictive optimal trees in emergency surgery risk (POTTER) calculator in emergency general surgery and emergency laparotomy patients. J Am Coll Surg. 2021;232(6):912–19.e1.

20. Bertsimas D, Dunn J, Velmahos GC, Kaafarani HMA. Surgical risk is not linear: derivation and validation of a novel, user-friendly, and machine-learning-based predictive optimal trees in emergency surgery risk (POTTER) calculator. Ann Surg. 2018;268(4):574–83.
21. El Moheb M, Gebran A, Maurer LR, et al. Artificial intelligence versus surgeon gestalt in predicting risk of emergency general surgery. J Trauma Acute Care Surg. 2023;95(4):565–72.
22. Morris MX, Fiocco D, Caneva T, et al. Current and future applications of artificial intelligence in surgery: implications for clinical practice and research. Front Surg. 2024;11:1393898.
23. Ferreres AR. Ethical and legal issues regarding artificial intelligence (AI) and management of surgical data. Eur J Surg Oncol. 2025;51(1):108279.

Nurse Support and Home Care Services for Older Surgical Patients: Models, Roles, and Future Perspectives

5

Belinda De Simone, Angelo Ferraro, Jury Ascolese, and Fausto Catena

5.1 Introduction

The global population is aging rapidly: by 2050, over 1.5 billion people will be aged 65 or older, with adults over 80 representing the fastest-growing age group worldwide [1]. In Europe, nearly 40% of surgical procedures are performed on patients aged 65 and over, and this figure is expected to rise as life expectancy increases and surgical indications expand to frail older adults [2].

Older surgical patients face significantly higher risks of adverse outcomes, including postoperative delirium, infections, prolonged immobility, loss of independence, and hospital readmission. According to a recent meta-analysis, frailty increases the risk of major postoperative complications by 2.5 times and mortality by 1.7 times [3]. Functional decline is frequently observed, with up to 30% of older patients losing the ability to perform activities of daily living (ADLs) after surgery [4].

The transition from hospital to home is particularly critical: it often occurs rapidly, especially in fast-track or Enhanced Recovery After Surgery (ERAS®)

B. De Simone (✉)
Department of Emergency Minimally Invasive Surgery, Trauma Hub Center, Bufalini Hospital, AUSL Romagna, Cesena, Italy

Department of Theoretical and Applied Sciences, eCampus University, Novedrate (CO), Italy
e-mail: desimone.belinda@gmail.com

A. Ferraro · J. Ascolese
General and Emergency Surgery Unit, Infermi Hospital, AUSL Romagna, Rimini, Italy
e-mail: angelo.ferraro@auslromagna.it; jury.ascolese@auslromagna.it

F. Catena
Department of Medical and Surgical Sciences, Alma Mater Studiorum University of Bologna, Bologna, Italy

P. Carcoforo, F. Catena (eds.), *Geriatric Surgery*, Updates in Surgery, https://doi.org/10.1007/978-3-032-24281-5_5

pathways, without sufficient time to establish effective discharge plans or train caregivers [5]. Studies show that poorly coordinated discharge increases the risk of readmission, inappropriate medication use, and caregiver burden [6, 7]. In this vulnerable phase, nursing-led transitional care programs and structured home care services have emerged as key strategies to support safe recovery, prevent complications, and promote autonomy in older adults.

This chapter examines the role of nurses in managing postoperative transitions and the models of home-based care implemented across healthcare systems. Drawing from national and international examples, it explores current practices, barriers, and opportunities for innovation, with special attention to caregiver support, geriatric assessment, and digital health integration.

5.2 The Role of Nurses in Transitional and Home Care

The hospital-to-home transition is a vulnerable phase for older surgical patients, who are at increased risk of care discontinuity, medication errors, and functional decline. In this context, nurses play a pivotal role as care coordinators, educators, and advocates for patients and their families. Their involvement is particularly relevant in systems where hospital stays are shorter and early discharge is the norm.

Nurse-led transitional care programs (TCPs) have been developed to support patients after hospital discharge. These programs typically include structured discharge planning, home visits or follow-up phone calls, medication reconciliation, caregiver education, and coordination with general practitioners and specialists. Evidence shows that such interventions improve satisfaction, enhance self-management, and reduce readmissions [8–15].

Recent meta-analyses have confirmed that nurse-driven transitional care can significantly reduce hospital readmission rates and improve quality of life, especially for older adults with multiple comorbidities [2, 3, 16]. For instance, in a randomized controlled trial of elderly patients undergoing cardiac surgery, those who received nurse-led transitional care experienced fewer postoperative complications, shorter readmissions, and better functional outcomes compared to those receiving standard care [17].

Nurses contribute not only to physical recovery but also to psychosocial well-being. Studies highlight the importance of culturally competent communication, emotional support, and health literacy coaching—particularly for patients from socioeconomically disadvantaged backgrounds [2, 9]. In critical care settings, nurse interventions targeting family members have also improved the perceived quality of communication and emotional support [18].

Moreover, the nursing role in transitional care is dynamic and multidimensional: it requires clinical judgment, technical skills, digital literacy (e.g., for teleconsultation and electronic care coordination), and a deep understanding of social determinants of health. Nurses are uniquely positioned to assess both medical and psychosocial needs, allowing them to tailor post-discharge plans to each patient's context.

Despite growing evidence of their effectiveness, nurse-led TCPs face challenges in scalability and standardization. Future research should focus on defining core components, identifying best practices across settings, and integrating digital tools into nurse workflows to enhance efficiency and patient engagement.

5.3 Home Care Services: Overview and National Models

Across Europe, home care has become a cornerstone of healthcare delivery for older adults, especially in the postoperative phase. Despite structural differences between countries, all national models share the goals of improving quality of life, reducing inappropriate hospitalizations, and promoting functional recovery in place. In this section, we present an overview of the most relevant home care structures in Italy, France, and the United Kingdom, focusing on their organization, workforce, and integration with hospital services, as summarized in Table 5.1.

5.3.1 Italy

In Italy, the national strategy for strengthening territorial care was formalized with Ministerial Decree 77/2022, within the framework of the National Recovery and Resilience Plan [19]. The reform introduced key elements such as Integrated Home

Table 5.1 Comparison of National Home Care Models (Italy—France—UK)

Feature	Italy	France	United Kingdom
Main programs	ADI, SAD, Community nurses	HAD, SSIAD, SPASAD	ICS, District nurses, Home First, Discharge to Assess
Coordination entity	ASLs	Hospital-authorized HAD units	NHS ICSs
Multidisciplinary teams	Yes (nurse, GP, therapist, social worker)	Yes	Yes
Clinical + Social support	Separate services (ADI vs SAD)	Integrated in SPASAD	Integrated via ICS and local authorities
Telemedicine integration	In development (as per PNRR)	Partial, depending on region	Broad, with structured remote care programs
Cost coverage	Publicly funded (regional variance possible)	Fully reimbursed by Assurance Maladie	Publicly funded through NHS and social care

ADI Assistenza Domiciliare Integrata/Integrated Home Care, *ASLs* Local Health Authorities, *GP* general practitioner, *HAD* Hospitalisation à Domicile/Hospital at Home, *ICS* Integrated Care System, *NHS* National Health Service, *PNRR* Piano Nazionale di Ripresa e Resilienza/Italy's National Recovery and Resilience Plan (post-COVID), *SAD* Servizio di Assistenza Domiciliare/Home Assistance Service, *SPASAD* Services Polyvalents d'Aide et de Soins à Domicile/Combined Home Assistance and Nursing Services, *SSIAD* Services de Soins Infirmiers à Domicile/Home Nursing Services

Care (ADI), Community Health Houses, Family and Community Nurses, and the reinforcement of telemedicine infrastructures.

ADI provides coordinated multidisciplinary services, including nursing, medical, and rehabilitative care, delivered directly at home for frail and non-self-sufficient individuals. It is managed by Local Health Authorities (ASLs) and aims to progressively reach up to 10% of the population aged 65 and older. The Servizio di Assistenza Domiciliare (SAD), provided by municipalities, complements clinical care with social assistance (e.g., hygiene, meals, personal support). These services are publicly funded and tailored to local needs.

5.3.2 France

The French model of home care is centered around Hospitalisation à Domicile (HAD), regulated by the Code de la Santé Publique. HAD allows hospital-level treatments to be delivered at home under the supervision of accredited hospital facilities, involving multidisciplinary teams [20].

Complementary services include the Services de Soins Infirmiers à Domicile (SSIAD), which provide nursing care for frail and chronically ill older adults, and the Services Polyvalents d'Aide et de Soins à Domicile (SPASAD) programs, which integrate nursing and social support. These systems are designed to ensure continuity of care between hospitals and community settings and are fully reimbursed by the national insurance system.

5.3.3 United Kingdom

In the UK, home care for older adults is embedded within the National Health Service (NHS) and delivered through Integrated Care Systems (ICS). The model is built around the concept of "Home First", which promotes early discharge and supports recovery in the patient's own home environment [21].

Key professionals include district nurses, who work closely with general practitioners and social care providers. Services are patient-centered, emphasizing multidisciplinary collaboration and personalized care planning. Recent developments have expanded the use of telehealth and community rehabilitation programs, particularly for patients with cancer, dementia, or multimorbidity. The Discharge to Assess model enables patients to complete clinical assessments and rehabilitation at home after early hospital discharge [22].

These models reflect a shared commitment to enhance home-based care for older adults, but also reveal variability in structure, access, and digital integration. While Italy is undergoing major reforms to decentralize care and standardize regional services [19], France leverages a hospital-led system with strong medical oversight [20]. The UK, in contrast, emphasizes early discharge and integrated community rehabilitation through NHS policy frameworks [21, 22].

5.4 Postoperative Rehabilitation at Home

Older surgical patients often face a prolonged and complex recovery process due to pre-existing frailty, sarcopenia, cognitive decline, and functional impairment. Postoperative rehabilitation at home is a crucial component of the recovery pathway, aiming to restore independence, prevent complications, and promote quality of life.

Rehabilitation in this setting is inherently multidisciplinary, involving nurses, physiotherapists, dietitians, occupational therapists, and general practitioners. It encompasses physical reconditioning, nutritional support, cognitive stimulation, and functional training, tailored to the patient's specific needs and home environment.

In Table 5.2 are summarized evidence-based models supporting home-based postoperative rehabilitation in older adults. Outcomes are drawn from representative studies and systematic reviews [23–29].

A key framework for planning individualized rehabilitation is the Comprehensive Geriatric Assessment (CGA). This multidimensional, interdisciplinary diagnostic process evaluates medical, functional, cognitive, nutritional, and social domains. It enables healthcare professionals to identify modifiable risk factors and personalize perioperative care plans [2, 3].

One of the main risk factors is sarcopenia, the progressive loss of muscle mass and strength, which is strongly associated with postoperative complications, longer hospital stays, and increased mortality [30]. Home-based programs that combine nutritional supplementation with resistance and aerobic training have shown promising results in reducing functional decline and readmissions [31].

Malnutrition is another prevalent issue in older adults. The Mini Nutritional Assessment (MNA) is widely used to screen for nutritional risk and guide dietary interventions. Malnourished patients may benefit from tailored nutrition plans with high-protein, micronutrient-rich diets, which support wound healing, immune function, and overall recovery [32].

Table 5.2 Postoperative Rehabilitation Models and Clinical Outcomes

Model/Approach	Main features	Clinical outcomes
Early supported discharge (ESD)	Shortened hospital stay; multidisciplinary home follow-up	↓ length of stay, ↑ patient satisfaction [23]
Hospital at home (HAD)	Acute care delivered at home; structured protocols; hospital-equivalent	↓ readmission and institutionalization rates [24]
Integrated transitional care	Structured handover between hospital and community services	Improved continuity, ↓ adverse events [25]
Nurse-led home rehabilitation	Home visits, patient education, wound care, functional recovery follow-up	↑ functional independence, ↓ complications [29]
Multidisciplinary case management	Geriatrician, nurse, physio, social worker coordination post-discharge	↓ caregiver burden, ↑ care coordination [26]
Digital rehabilitation tools	Wearables, apps, and remote monitoring tools for rehab and symptom tracking	↑ adherence, ↓ hospital revisits in frail elderly [27]

Cognitive dysfunction, including mild cognitive impairment or dementia, may interfere with rehabilitation adherence, self-care, and communication. The Mini Mental State Examination (MMSE) is commonly used to assess cognitive status in the context of CGA. Cognitive training programs, including memory exercises and problem-solving tasks, have been shown to reduce the risk of postoperative cognitive decline [33].

Functional status is equally critical: tools like the Barthel Index are used to assess patients' ability to perform ADLs. Older adults with impaired mobility or recent falls may require environmental adaptations (e.g., grab bars, walking aids) or caregiver support during early ambulation [34]. Home-based physiotherapy, when integrated into daily routines, is effective in maintaining mobility and preventing deconditioning.

In many countries, including Italy, France, and the UK, the implementation of structured models such as Early Supported Discharge (ESD) and HAD has shown favorable outcomes in reducing complications, improving functional recovery, and shortening the length of hospital stay. These approaches enable patients to return home earlier while still receiving multidisciplinary follow-up and therapeutic interventions.

The literature supports the effectiveness of nurse-led and transitional care models in enhancing medication adherence, empowering caregivers, and facilitating coordination with primary care physicians [23, 25]. The HAD model, in particular, offers hospital-level care at home, including IV therapies and monitoring, demonstrating comparable or superior outcomes in terms of patient satisfaction and readmission rates [26].

In the orthopedic field, especially following hip fracture surgery, home-based rehabilitation has proven effective in improving mobility, balance, and overall independence. Patient adherence and the presence of an engaged caregiver remain key success factors [27–29].

The ERAS® protocol also contributes to the shift toward early discharge and home recovery [5]. Its structured follow-up and interdisciplinary coordination are aligned with CGA principles, emphasizing personalized goals and functional optimization [35].

Evidence suggests that these models are most effective in older adults who are hemodynamically stable, live in safe home environments, and benefit from caregiver support. Surgical indications that lend themselves well to home-based recovery include low- to moderate-complexity abdominal procedures, orthopedic surgeries, and selected cardiothoracic cases, particularly in clinically stable chronic patients [36, 37].

Nonetheless, broader implementation remains challenging due to variability in local resources, caregiver availability, staff training, information sharing between hospital and community, and associated costs. Continued research is needed to harmonize these models and improve their scalability in light of demographic aging.

The nurse plays a central role in this process. From the preoperative phase, nurses are involved in educating patients, coordinating CGA-based assessments, and identifying high-risk individuals. Postoperatively, they monitor recovery, provide wound and medication management, and liaise with other professionals to ensure rehabilitation goals are met.

Although the implementation of CGA in routine surgical practice may be complex, its benefits in risk stratification, care planning, and outcome prediction justify broader adoption. Home rehabilitation guided by CGA not only improves functional outcomes but also reduces caregiver burden and healthcare costs [38, 39].

5.5 Comprehensive Geriatric Assessment (CGA) and Home Care Planning

CGA is a multidimensional, multidisciplinary evaluation process designed to assess the medical, psychological, functional, and social capabilities of older adults. Within the surgical context, CGA has emerged as a cornerstone of perioperative planning, especially for tailoring home-based recovery interventions and reducing avoidable complications [39].

Frailty, defined as a multi-system physiological decline that heightens vulnerability to stressors such as surgery, is often associated with adverse postoperative outcomes. Its frequent co-occurrence with cognitive impairment contributes to increased rates of postoperative delirium, which itself is linked to higher morbidity, prolonged hospital stays, and increased mortality [40].

CGA supports a coordinated care model that spans preoperative, perioperative, and post-discharge phases. It enables the multidisciplinary team, including geriatricians, anesthesiologists, surgeons, geriatric nurses, physiotherapists, occupational therapists, and dietitians, to formulate integrated, personalized care plans. These plans often include tailored exercise protocols, nutrition therapy, medication adjustments, or rehabilitation strategies that are reassessed and adapted over time [39, 41].

CGA is guided by age-friendly care principles such as: (1) understanding what matters most to the patient, (2) managing multi-complexity, (3) optimizing medication, (4) assessing mentation, and (5) ensuring mobility. These principles shape both the content of the assessment and the goals of the care plan [41, 42].

When performed preoperatively, CGA facilitates early involvement of nurses and allied professionals. Nurses typically initiate contact to gather medication lists, assess fall risk, and administer tools such as the MNA and MMSE [41]. This proactive approach is key to designing a realistic, risk-based discharge plan that includes home rehabilitation and community support.

However, implementing CGA in emergency surgical settings poses unique challenges. Critically ill patients may present with hemodynamic instability and atypical clinical signs, and time constraints often limit the capacity to assemble full multidisciplinary teams. In these cases, emergency physicians, surgeons and anesthesiologists must make rapid yet ethically grounded decisions. Shared decision-making, realistic medicine principles, and frailty screening tools such as the Rockwood Clinical Frailty Scale can guide treatment escalation plans, even in the absence of geriatric specialists [43] (Fig. 5.1).

Key Principles for Applying Comprehensive Geriatric Assessment (CGA) in Emergency Surgical Settings

1. **Initial Evaluation**

- Obtain a comprehensive history: comorbidities, functional status, mobility, mental health, and living situation
- Assess frailty using the Rockwood Clinical Frailty Scale
- Screen for delirium with validated tools (e.g., 4AT, CAM)

2. **Acute Medical Management**

- Correct physiological derangements (fluids, electrolytes, pain)
- Consider polypharmacy and age-related pharmacokinetics in treatment

3. **Decision-Making and Escalation Planning**

- Engage patients, caregivers and family members in shared decisions
- Define and document ceilings of care using appropriate legal frameworks
- Respect patient values, pre-existing directives, and ethical considerations

4. **Postoperative CGA and Follow-Up**

- Involve geriatricians and multidisciplinary teams as soon as possible in the postoperative care
- Activate home-based rehabilitation and transitional care planning
- Ensure nurse-led coordination and continuity with primary care

When no preoperative frailty team is available, emergency surgeons and anesthesiologists should apply these CGA-aligned principles to improve patient outcomes and minimize complications.

Fig. 5.1 Comprehensive Geriatric Assessment principles for emergency surgical patients

In literature, the Elder-Friendly Approaches to the Surgical Environment (EASE) model have shown that CGA-inspired, elder-friendly interventions can reduce major in-hospital complications, lower mortality, and shorten length of stay. Similarly, the Acute Care for the Elderly (ACE) model promotes interdisciplinary care, early rehabilitation, and functional preservation, all of which are associated with improved patient outcomes and higher rates of discharge to home rather than institutional settings [44, 45].

National guidelines now recommend assessing frailty and cognitive status for all patients aged ≥65 undergoing surgery, whether elective or emergent—and emphasize the need to involve geriatricians pre- or postoperatively whenever possible.

During the pre-discharge phase, CGA findings are translated into practical home care actions. For example:

- Patients with impaired mobility may require scheduled home physiotherapy.
- Malnourished patients may need dietitian follow-up and assistance with meal preparation.
- Those with mild cognitive deficits may benefit from telemonitoring, caregiver training, or simplified medication regimens.

CGA also guides the stratification of post-discharge risk, helping to determine whether patients are candidates for early supported discharge, HAD models, or intermediate care. The role of the nurse case manager is central in ensuring continuity of care through coordination with general practitioners, home care services, and informal caregivers [46].

Additionally, CGA allows for shared decision-making: patients and families are informed of potential risks and participate in developing realistic care goals. This is particularly relevant for patients with advanced frailty, for whom a palliative approach or reduced therapeutic intensity may be appropriate [46].

Despite its recognized utility, CGA is not yet systematically implemented in all surgical pathways. Barriers include time constraints, lack of interdisciplinary coordination, and variability in assessment tools. However, increasing evidence supports its value in reducing readmissions, improving functional outcomes, and enhancing patient and caregiver satisfaction [41, 46].

In summary, CGA is not only an assessment tool but a strategic platform for integrating medical, social, and functional domains into home care planning. Nurses, as coordinators and interpreters of the CGA, play a critical role in ensuring that its insights translate into individualized, effective post-discharge care.

5.6 Caregiver Support and Education

Family caregivers, whether spouses, children, friends, or neighbors, are often the backbone of postoperative care for older adults, particularly after early hospital discharge. As healthcare systems increasingly rely on home-based recovery, the complexity, intensity, and duration of informal caregiving continue to grow. Nurses play a pivotal role in educating, supporting, and empowering caregivers to manage their responsibilities safely and confidently [47, 48].

In the surgical setting, caregivers must often handle tasks such as medication administration, wound care, hygiene, mobility assistance, communication with professionals, and symptom monitoring. Despite this, many receive minimal training or support. A nurse-led therapeutic education program can significantly improve caregiver preparedness and reduce preventable complications.

Carrillo et al. [48] evaluated a structured intervention for caregivers of cancer surgery patients. It included:

- Group sessions at hospital admission to assess knowledge and prepare for discharge,
- Hands-on workshops with devices and medication management,
- Distribution of educational materials,
- Individual counseling on fears, support networks, and coping mechanisms,
- Weekly phone follow-ups for 4 weeks post-discharge.

This intervention improved caregiver competence, reduced anxiety, and enhanced continuity of care.

Other studies emphasize that caregiver strain is not only functional but also emotional and social. According to a synthesis by Schultz et al. [49], the main risk factors for caregiver distress include:

- Low income or educational level,
- Advanced age and female gender,
- Intense caregiving load (>100 hours/month),
- Poor health status of the patient (e.g., dementia),
- Lack of support networks,
- Perceived lack of choice in taking on the caregiver role,
- Difficult home environments (e.g., unsafe layout, clutter).

To address these challenges, multicomponent support strategies are recommended:

- Tailored education on care tasks, symptoms, and red flags,
- Psychological support and stress coping programs (e.g., mindfulness, peer support),
- Technology-based tools for teleassistance and guided decision-making,
- Respite care services to provide temporary relief from caregiving,
- Adaptive communication strategies based on caregiver literacy and learning style.

Nurses are central to delivering these interventions. Their empathy, communication skills, and clinical insight allow them to identify overwhelmed caregivers early and offer customized support. Furthermore, integrating caregiver assessment into the hospital discharge process helps proactively flag at-risk families and initiate supportive services [47–49].

Ultimately, supporting caregivers is not optional, it is a clinical, ethical, and systemic necessity in modern postoperative care. When caregivers are informed, confident, and supported, outcomes improve for everyone: the patient, the family, and the healthcare system.

5.7 Technology-Enhanced Home Care

The integration of digital tools into home care is reshaping the way postoperative support is delivered to older adults. Known collectively as eHealth, these interventions include telemedicine, remote monitoring, video consultations, and mobile applications designed to enhance patient self-management and care coordination [50]. According to the World Health Organization, eHealth refers to the "use of information and communication technologies for health" and has become increasingly relevant in postoperative pathways, especially for frail or homebound individuals [51].

Older adults, however, face specific barriers in adopting technology: limited digital literacy, sensory impairments, cognitive challenges, and anxiety related to unfamiliar tools. Despite these obstacles, evidence suggests that when appropriately designed and supported, digital interventions can reduce readmissions, identify complications early, and enhance quality of life [52, 53].

Examples of digital tools used in postoperative care include:

- Teleconsultations via video platforms (Zoom®, Teams®) for wound evaluation, education, and follow-up,
- Mobile applications for symptom tracking, medication reminders, and exercise programs,
- Wearable sensors (e.g., smartwatches) that monitor vital signs, mobility, or sleep quality,
- Automated alerts for abnormal parameters that notify nurses or physicians in real time.

The Digital Health Innovation (DHI) model emphasizes the use of mobile and wireless technologies to improve health system efficiency and patient outcomes. These systems allow patients to self-report symptoms, receive personalized feedback, and maintain communication with healthcare providers from home [52, 53]. For nurses, DHI provides tools to monitor clinical trends, triage symptoms, and prioritize visits (Box 5.1).

Box 5.1 Clinical Vignette

Mr. B., an 82-year-old patient discharged after elective colorectal surgery, was enrolled in a telemonitoring program coordinated by the hospital's nurse case manager. He and his daughter were trained to use a tablet-based app to record daily temperature, pain levels, and wound images. During the second week at home, the nurse received an automatic alert triggered by a reported low-grade fever and delayed wound healing. A video consultation was scheduled the same day, during which mild erythema was observed. The nurse contacted the surgical team and adjusted the wound care plan. This early intervention prevented progression to infection and avoided readmission.

Nevertheless, the success of technology-enhanced care depends on training, accessibility, and human support. Nurses play a crucial role in:

- Teaching patients and caregivers how to use devices,
- Interpreting data and acting on alerts,
- Adjusting care plans based on remote observations,
- Ensuring digital equity by addressing usability and literacy gaps.

Designing user-friendly systems is essential. Key features that improve usability for older adults include:

- Large fonts and icons,
- Clear color coding,
- Simple navigation,
- Availability of non-digital alternatives (e.g., printed instructions or caregiver interfaces).

Digital solutions also offer psychosocial benefits: they reduce travel burdens, promote patient autonomy, and help mitigate social isolation, particularly relevant for patients with limited mobility or distant caregivers. However, most of the evidence comes from high-income countries, and accessibility remains a global concern.

In conclusion, while digital tools are not a substitute for human care, they can enhance safety, efficiency, and personalization of home care when guided by trained professionals. Nurses are not only clinical caregivers but also digital mediators who can bridge the gap between innovation and patient-centered care.

5.8 Challenges and Barriers

While nurse-led home care and transitional models offer clear benefits for older surgical patients, their widespread implementation still faces several challenges, many of which are systemic, structural, and sociocultural.

A major limitation is the shortage of nurses trained in geriatric care and transitional coordination. In many systems, nursing staff are already stretched thin by hospital and community workloads. The skillset required to manage frail elderly patients, such as conducting CGA-informed planning, coordinating multidisciplinary care, and supporting caregivers, requires specific training that is not yet universally available [2, 3].

Another critical issue is the fragmentation between hospital-based and community-based services. Discharge planning often remains unstructured, with poor communication between hospital physicians, general practitioners, and home care providers. Without shared digital records or interoperable platforms, nurses may lack access to essential information about surgery, medications, or risk status, resulting in safety gaps and inefficiencies [50].

Even when digital systems are available, technological barriers persist, especially for the elderly. Limited familiarity with smartphones, sensory impairments, and low digital literacy can undermine the effectiveness of eHealth tools [52]. Moreover, many platforms are not designed with older users in mind, leading to usability problems and inequitable access. Nurses themselves may not receive adequate digital training, reducing confidence in using remote monitoring systems or video consultations.

Caregivers, too, often lack the knowledge or confidence to manage postoperative needs. While nurse-led education programs have proven effective [47, 48], they are not consistently offered. When caregivers feel unprepared or unsupported, their burden increases, raising the risk of stress, burnout, and poor adherence to follow-up plans [49, 54].

Geographical and socioeconomic disparities also contribute to unequal access to home care services. In rural or underserved areas, home visits may be logistically difficult, and families may struggle with out-of-pocket expenses for essential items such as dressings, mobility aids, or caregiver support. These gaps reflect broader equity challenges in healthcare delivery.

Finally, institutional culture and policy inertia may limit progress. In some settings, home care is still perceived as "ancillary" or less clinical. Nurse-led models may lack recognition or formal support, which restricts investment, training opportunities, and integration into surgical pathways.

In summary, to fully unlock the potential of home-based recovery and transitional care, healthcare systems must overcome not only logistical and workforce challenges, but also cultural and digital divides. Empowering nurses, integrating services, and investing in equitable access will be essential steps toward safer, more personalized care for older surgical patients.

5.9 Future Directions and Policy Implications

As populations continue to age and the complexity of surgical patients increases, nurse-led home care will play an ever more central role in ensuring safe recovery, minimizing institutional dependency, and improving patient-centered outcomes. To achieve this, healthcare systems must move beyond isolated pilot programs and toward system-wide transformation.

In some healthcare systems, particularly in the UK, virtual wards (VWs) have emerged as innovative models of care that allow patients to receive hospital-level treatment at home, supported by remote monitoring technologies and daily clinical oversight. While not all virtual wards are nurse-led, many rely heavily on community nurses, advanced nurse practitioners, and case managers to coordinate care, monitor parameters, and escalate treatment when needed [15].

In the context of surgical recovery and frail older patients, VWs may support early discharge by providing structured follow-up, symptom monitoring, and remote access to clinicians. Technologies used include pulse oximeters, digital blood pressure monitors, tablet-based surveys, and teleconsultation platforms. Nurse involvement is crucial to assess signs of deterioration, ensure adherence to rehabilitation protocols, and provide psychosocial support [55].

Evidence suggests that VWs can reduce emergency readmissions, improve patient satisfaction, and free up hospital beds. However, issues of digital equity, interoperability, and clinical responsibility boundaries remain open challenges [15, 55]. In countries like Italy and France, integrating VW principles within existing HAD or ADI models could represent a strategic evolution toward digitally enabled home care.

The future of postoperative care for older adults lies in personalized, proactive, and integrated models, where home becomes the new clinical frontier. This vision requires investment, training, and a redefinition of roles, particularly for nurses, who are uniquely positioned to lead this transition.

The mandatory actions to establish the evolution of care for geriatric surgical patients are:

- **Strengthening the nursing workforce**. Nurses must be equipped with specialized training in geriatrics, transitional care, digital health, and care coordination. National curricula should include modules on frailty assessment, caregiver support, and discharge planning. Establishing the role of nurse case managers or community nurse specialists in postoperative pathways can improve continuity, reduce readmissions, and increase patient satisfaction. These roles should be formally recognized, adequately funded, and included in national staffing plans.
- **Integrating services and information systems**. True continuity of care requires interoperable digital systems that allow seamless communication between hospitals, primary care providers, and home care teams. Nurses must have access to discharge summaries, medication changes, risk assessments, and follow-up plans, ideally in real time. Policy-makers should incentivize shared care platforms, formal discharge protocols, and integrated transition teams that include nurses, general practitioners, physiotherapists, and social workers.
- **Making digital health work for older adults**. To ensure equitable access, technology must be adapted to older patients, not the other way around. This includes user-centered design, simplified interfaces, visual accessibility, and availability of hybrid (digital + human) options. Nurses should receive continuous training in telemedicine, mobile health, and wearable data interpretation. Policy-makers should support the scaling of successful digital health pilots, with special attention to inclusion, usability, and data privacy.
- **Supporting family caregivers as co-providers**. Caregivers should be recognized as essential partners in the recovery process. Structured education programs, psychosocial support, and respite services must be embedded in surgical discharge pathways. National health policies should include caregiver assessment tools, formal referral pathways, and funding for caregiver-inclusive programs, particularly in cases of complex or long-term recovery.

- **Reframing home care as "Essential Care"**. Too often, home care is still perceived as ancillary or "non-urgent." The COVID-19 pandemic demonstrated that decentralized, flexible, and home-based models are not only viable, they are essential. Going forward, postoperative care must be designed with the home setting in mind from the start.
- This includes:
  - Implementing CGA-based pathways as standard in older surgical patients,
  - Defining minimum care packages for home follow-up,
  - Recognizing home care outcomes (e.g., functional recovery, caregiver burden) as key quality indicators.

Achieving these goals will require political will, professional leadership, and cross-sector collaboration. Hospitals must open to continuity-based logic. Communities must be empowered. Nurses must be trusted and supported.

By bridging innovation with equity, and professionalism with compassion, we can shape a postoperative care system where aging, surgery, and recovery are no longer points of rupture but part of a seamless, supported life journey.

5.9.1 Key Operational Recommendations for Implementation of Nurse Support and Home Care Services in Clinical Practice

Based on the findings and models discussed in this chapter, we propose the following priorities for implementation:

1. Establish nurse-led transitional care teams within surgical pathways for older patients.
2. Incorporate CGA as a standard step in preoperative assessment for frail adults.
3. Fund structured education programs for caregivers, led by trained nurses.
4. Integrate interoperable digital platforms across hospital and community services.
5. Train nurses in digital health tools, including remote monitoring and teleconsultation.
6. Ensure user-friendly design in eHealth tools to accommodate older adults.
7. Include home care metrics (functional status, caregiver strain, readmission) in quality indicators.
8. Recognize and finance the role of nurse case managers or community liaison nurses.
9. Invest in rural and underserved areas to reduce inequality in access to home care.
10. Redefine home care as essential, integrating it structurally into postoperative protocols.

5.10 Conclusion

Older adults undergoing surgery represent a vulnerable and growing population, often requiring complex and prolonged recovery beyond hospital discharge. This chapter has highlighted the central role of nurses and home care services in ensuring safe, effective, and personalized postoperative pathways for frail patients.

From transitional care coordination to CGA-informed planning, caregiver education, and the integration of digital tools, nurses are uniquely positioned to bridge clinical care with the realities of patients' daily lives. International models, despite structural differences, converge on a shared recognition: the home is not the end point of care, but a critical care setting in itself.

To deliver on this promise, healthcare systems must invest in:

- The training and empowerment of nursing professionals,
- The integration of hospital and community services,
- The scaling of inclusive digital innovations,
- The support of informal caregivers as core actors in recovery.

This is not merely a matter of efficiency or cost, it is a question of dignity, safety, and human-centered care.

Redesigning surgical recovery with the home in mind, and with nurses at the center, is not just a future vision, it is an actionable imperative. By translating knowledge into structure, and compassion into strategy, we can ensure that even after surgery, our most vulnerable patients are never left alone at the edge of the system, but supported, respected, and cared for, where it matters most.

References

1. World Health Organization. Decade of healthy ageing [Internet]. World Health Organization; 2020 [cited 2025 Sept 15]. Available from: https://apps.who.int/gb/ebwha/pdf_files/WHA73/A73_INF2-en.pdf.
2. Theodorakis N, Nikolaou M, Hitas C, et al. Comprehensive peri-operative risk assessment and management of geriatric patients. Diagnostics (Basel). 2024;14(19):2153.
3. Chen L, Zong W, Luo M, Yu H. The impact of comprehensive geriatric assessment on post-operative outcomes in elderly surgery: a systematic review and meta-analysis. PLoS One. 2024;19(8):e0306308.
4. Janssen TL, Lodder P, de Vries J, et al. Caregiver strain on informal caregivers when providing care for older patients undergoing major abdominal surgery: a longitudinal prospective cohort study. BMC Geriatr. 2020;20(1):178.
5. ERAS® Society. Guidelines [Internet]. ERAS® Society; 2025 [cited 2025 Sept 15]. Available from: https://erassociety.org/guidelines/.
6. Kripalani S, Theobald CN, Anctil B, Vasilevskis EE. Reducing hospital readmission rates: current strategies and future directions. Annu Rev Med. 2014;65:471–85.
7. Dhaliwal JS, Dang AK. Reducing hospital readmissions. In: StatPearls [Internet]. Treasure Island: StatPearls Publishing; 2025.

8. Sakashita C, Endo E, Ota E, Oku H. Effectiveness of nurse-led transitional care interventions for adult patients discharged from acute care hospitals: a systematic review and meta-analysis. BMC Nurs. 2025;24(1):379.
9. Berthelsen C, Møller N, Bunkenborg G. Transitional care model for older adults with multiple chronic conditions: an evaluation of benefits utilising an umbrella review. J Clin Nurs. 2024;33(2):481–96.
10. McParland C, Johnston B, Cooper M. A mixed-methods systematic review of nurse-led interventions for people with multimorbidity. J Adv Nurs. 2022;78(12):3930–51.
11. Conneely M, Leahy S, Dore L, et al. The effectiveness of interventions to reduce adverse outcomes among older adults following emergency department discharge: umbrella review. BMC Geriatr. 2022;22(1):462.
12. Fønss Rasmussen L, Grode LB, Lange J, et al. Impact of transitional care interventions on hospital readmissions in older medical patients: a systematic review. BMJ Open. 2021;11(1):e040057.
13. Birtwell K, Planner C, Hodkinson A, et al. Transitional care interventions for older residents of long-term care facilities: a systematic review and meta-analysis. JAMA Netw Open. 2022;5(5):e2210192.
14. Marini G, Longhini J, Ambrosi E, et al. Transitional care interventions in improving patient and caregiver outcomes after discharge: a scoping review. Healthcare (Basel). 2025;13(3):312.
15. Norman G, Bennett P, Vardy ERLC. Virtual wards: a rapid evidence synthesis and implications for the care of older people. Age Ageing. 2023;52(1):afac319.
16. Li M, Li Y, Meng Q, et al. Effects of nurse-led transitional care interventions for patients with heart failure on healthcare utilization: a meta-analysis of randomized controlled trials. PLoS One. 2021;16(12):e0261300.
17. Coskun S, Duygulu S. The effects of nurse led transitional care model on elderly patients undergoing open heart surgery: a randomized controlled trial. Eur J Cardiovasc Nurs. 2022;21(1):46–55.
18. Naef R, Jeitziner MM, Riguzzi M, et al. Nurse-led family support intervention for families of critically ill patients: the FICUS cluster randomized clinical trial. JAMA Intern Med. 2025;185(9):1138–49.
19. Ministero della Salute. Decreto ministeriale 23 maggio 2022, n. 77. Modelli e standard per lo sviluppo dell'assistenza territoriale nel Servizio sanitario nazionale. Gazzetta Ufficiale, Serie Generale, n. 144 del 22-06-2022.
20. Ministère de la Santé et de la Prévention. Hospitalisation à domicile (HAD) et services de soins infirmiers à domicile (SSIAD). République Française. 2019;
21. NHS England. The NHS long term plan. National Health Service; 2018.
22. NHS. NHS discharge to assess model 2021/22. National Health Service; 2021.
23. Jack BW, Chetty VK, Anthony D, et al. A reengineered hospital discharge program to decrease rehospitalization: a randomized trial. Ann Intern Med. 2009;150(3):178–87.
24. Leff B, Burton L, Mader SL, et al. Hospital at home: feasibility and outcomes of a program to provide hospital-level care at home for acutely ill older patients. Ann Intern Med. 2005;143(11):798–808.
25. Coleman EA, Smith JD, Frank JC, et al. Preparing patients and caregivers to participate in care delivered across settings: the care transitions intervention. J Am Geriatr Soc. 2004;52(11):1817–25.
26. Edgar K, Iliffe S, Doll HA, et al. Admission avoidance hospital at home. Cochrane Database Syst Rev. 2024;3(3):CD007491.
27. Wu D, Zhu X, Zhang S. Effect of home-based rehabilitation for hip fracture: a meta-analysis of randomized controlled trials. J Rehabil Med. 2018;50(6):481–6.
28. Magaziner J, Mangione KK, Orwig D, et al. Effect of a multicomponent home-based physical therapy intervention on ambulation after hip fracture in older adults: the CAP randomized clinical trial. JAMA. 2019;322(10):946–56.

29. Fairhall NJ, Dyer SM, Mak JC, et al. Interventions for improving mobility after hip fracture surgery in adults. Cochrane Database Syst Rev. 2022;9(9):CD001704.
30. Knoedler S, Schliermann R, Knoedler L, et al. Impact of sarcopenia on outcomes in surgical patients: a systematic review and meta-analysis. Int J Surg. 2023;109(12):4238–62.
31. Özdemir R, Yaman F. An investigation into the effects of frailty and sarcopenia on postoperative anesthesia recovery and complications among geriatric patients undergoing colorectal malignancy surgery. Medicina (Kaunas). 2025;61(6):969.
32. Millrose M, Schmidt W, Krickl J, et al. Influence of malnutrition on outcome after hip fractures in older patients. J Pers Med. 2023;13(1):109.
33. Zhao L, Guo Y, Zhou X, et al. Preoperative cognitive training improves postoperative cognitive function: a meta-analysis and systematic review of randomized controlled trials. Front Neurol. 2024;14:1293153.
34. Saisana M. Barthel index. In: Michalos AC, editor. Encyclopedia of quality of life and well-being research. Dordrecht: Springer; 2014.
35. Ljungqvist O, Scott M, Fearon KC. Enhanced recovery after surgery: a review. JAMA Surg. 2017;152(3):292–8.
36. Shepperd S, Iliffe S, Doll HA, et al. Admission avoidance hospital at home. Cochrane Database Syst Rev. 2016;9(9):CD007491.
37. Gonçalves-Bradley DC, Iliffe S, Doll HA, et al. Early discharge hospital at home. Cochrane Database Syst Rev. 2017;6(6):CD000356.
38. Campbell AJ, Buchner DM. Unstable disability and the fluctuations of frailty. Age Ageing. 1997;26(4):315–8.
39. Parker SG, McCue P, Phelps K, et al. What is Comprehensive Geriatric Assessment (CGA)? An umbrella review. Age Ageing. 2018;47(1):149–55.
40. Panayi AC, Orkaby AR, Sakthivel D, et al. Impact of frailty on outcomes in surgical patients: a systematic review and meta-analysis. Am J Surg. 2019;218(2):393–400.
41. British Geriatrics Society Comprehensive Geriatric Assessment toolkit for primary care practitioners [Internet]. British Geriatrics Society; 2019 [cited 2025 Sept 15]. Available from: https://www.bgs.org.uk/sites/default/files/content/resources/files/2019-03-12/CGA%20Toolkit%20for%20Primary%20Care%20Practitioners_0.pdf.
42. Van Remoortel H, Laermans J, Avau B, et al. Effectiveness of iron supplementation with or without erythropoiesis-stimulating agents on red blood cell utilization in patients with preoperative anaemia undergoing elective surgery: a systematic review and meta-analysis. Transfus Med Rev. 2021;35(2):103–24.
43. De Simone B, Dhesi JK, Hoffman MR, et al. Geriatric surgical patients: is it possible to implement the comprehensive geriatric assessment in the emergency setting? Discov Health Systems. 2023;2:13.
44. Khadaroo RG, Warkentin LM, Wagg AS, et al. Clinical effectiveness of the elder-friendly approaches to the surgical environment initiative in emergency general surgery. JAMA Surg. 2020;155(4):e196021.
45. Fox MT, Persaud M, Maimets I, et al. Effectiveness of acute geriatric unit care using acute care for elders components: a systematic review and meta-analysis. J Am Geriatr Soc. 2012;60(12):2237–45.
46. British Geriatrics Society. Comprehensive Geriatric Assessment (CGA) hub [Internet]. British Geriatrics Society [cited 2025 Sept 15]. Available from: https://www.bgs.org.uk/CGA.
47. Carrillo GM, Laguna M, Gómez OJ, et al. Effect of an educational intervention for family caregivers of individuals with cancer in surgery. Enfermería Glob. 2021;61
48. Carrillo GM, Mesa ML, Burbano DV. Skills required in the care of cancer patients who undergo surgery in the hospital-home transition. J Cancer Educ. 2022;37(5):1364–71.
49. Schulz R, Beach SR, Czaja SJ, et al. Family caregiving for older adults. Annu Rev Psychol. 2020;71:635–59.

50. Jonker LT, Haveman ME, de Bock GH, et al. Feasibility of perioperative eHealth interventions for older surgical patients: a systematic review. J Am Med Dir Assoc. 2020;21(12):1844–51.e2.
51. World Health Organization. Global strategy on digital health 2020-2025 [Internet]. World Health Organization; 2021 [cited 2025 Sept 15]. Available from: https://www.who.int/docs/default-source/documents/gs4dhdaa2a9f352b0445bafbc79ca799dce4d.pdf.
52. Knight SR, Ng N, Tsanas A, et al. Mobile devices and wearable technology for measuring patient outcomes after surgery: a systematic review. NPJ Digit Med. 2021;4(1):157.
53. Wu X, Freeman S, Miyagi M, et al. Comprehensive geriatric assessment in the era of telemedicine. Geriatr Gerontol Int. 2024;24(Suppl 1):67–73.
54. OECD. Who cares? Attracting and retaining care workers for the elderly [Internet]. OECD Health Policy Studies, 2020. OECD Publishing, Paris [cited 2025 Sept 15]. Available from: https://doi.org/10.1787/92c0ef68-en.OECD.
55. Sunny T, Ravichandran N, Broughan J, et al. Practitioners' perspectives on implementation of acute virtual wards: a scoping review. PLOS Digit Health. 2025;4(5):e0000858.

Fast-Track and ERAS®

6

Antonio Crucitti, Pasquina M. C. Tomaiuolo, Giada Di Flumeri, Giuseppe Pedullà, Paolo Mirco, Francesco Sionne, Enrico Coletta, and Andrea Mazzari

6.1 Introduction

Operating rooms are increasingly open to the elderly: surgical procedures performed on those over 65 have skyrocketed, resulting in a veritable boom. According to the latest data, these surgeries account for 900,000 per year in Italy (out of a total of two million procedures), including at least 20,000 cardiac surgeries. These numbers are set to grow further, with overall surgical procedures expected to increase by 30% by 2030 and the number of elderly patients projected to rise by 50% [1].

This scenario, while highlighting a general improvement in the physical endurance of the elderly, also poses a cost problem for the Italian National Health Service (NHS). The exponential increase in surgeries in elderly patients "can be explained by three factors: first, the growing population of people over 65 due to longer life expectancy; second, the improved general condition of the elderly, in terms of both strength/physical fitness and psychological well-being; and third, the availability of increasingly safe and refined surgical techniques, which makes it possible to operate even on those most at risk" [1].

Reducing the resources required to manage surgical patients is important, as is allocating new resources to treat chronic diseases (cardiovascular diseases, diabetes, neurologic disorders, cancer, etc). This is particularly true for this subgroup of patients.

A further consideration concerns the heterogeneity of the elderly population: chronological age alone does not provide an adequate description of surgical risk. A 70-year-old marathon runner and a sedentary 70-year-old with advanced diabetes represent two completely different clinical scenarios. Therefore, the concept of "biological age" is increasingly being emphasized. Biological age integrates frailty,

A. Crucitti (✉) · P. M. C. Tomaiuolo · G. Di Flumeri · G. Pedullà · P. Mirco
F. Sionne · E. Coletta · A. Mazzari
General and Mininvasive Surgery Unit, Cristo Re Hospital, Rome, Italy
e-mail: antonio.crucitti@unicatt.it

P. Carcoforo, F. Catena (eds.), *Geriatric Surgery*, Updates in Surgery,
https://doi.org/10.1007/978-3-032-24281-5_6

functional status, comorbidities, and cognitive performance into a broader measure of resilience to surgical stress. Enhanced Recovery After Surgery (ERAS®), by standardizing care and anticipating complications, is particularly well suited to address this variability.

Another relevant factor is the psychosocial dimension of aging. Elderly patients undergoing surgery often experience anxiety, fear of losing independence, and depression. These aspects can negatively influence postoperative recovery. Incorporating psychological support, structured patient education, and the involvement of caregivers into ERAS® pathways is therefore crucial to maximize adherence and outcomes.

The advent of fast-track protocols (ERAS®) has, in addition providing to clear clinical advantages, significantly reduced these increasing costs. ERAS® is widely recognized as a multimodal perioperative management strategy following major surgery. The introduction of fast-track protocols represents a significant change in perioperative management, integrating recent advances in recovery practices and new evidence from the literature, with a multidisciplinary approach throughout the entire recovery period. ERAS® is also a multidisciplinary approach consisting of a series of evidence-based perioperative interventions, aimed at preserving immune function and enhancing recovery. Hospitalization and surgery always affect normal homeostasis; this process is known as the "surgical stress response" and involves both the immune and neuro-endocrine systems. The ERAS® program, applied to major surgery, is well known to reduce morbidity (50%), hospitalization (30%), and costs, while improving short-term outcomes and minimizing the surgical stress response caused by injury.

This multimodal approach to recovery was first outlined by a Danish surgeon, Henrik Kehlet, in 1995 for colonic resections [2]; later this approach developed into what is now known as ERAS®. The process was initially applied only to colorectal surgery but has since been adopted across many different surgical specialties, including major operations. As shown by recent meta-analyses, this protocol is associated with a significantly reduced risk of complications and shorter hospitalization. The ERAS® pathway has been proven to be beneficial for patients and should now be considered the standard of care in colorectal surgery.

Moreover, many recent studies [3] have demonstrated a correlation between adherence to the items of the enhanced recovery protocol and improved outcomes. However, the question remains whether we can obtain the same results when applying ERAS® to older patients.

To answer this question, we first need to define "older patients". In the current literature, the cutoff varies, and is often set at age 70 or above. Elderly patients have higher levels of comorbidity, frailty, and social care requirements and reduced stress reactions. Therefore, ERAS® protocols should be the ideal care pathway in this subgroup of patients, as they aim to minimize stress on vulnerable organs. ERAS® represents a philosophy of care, and fast-track programs are changing the way modern surgical care is delivered. For colorectal cancer, the Italian Medical Oncology Association (AIOM) [4] reported in 2021 an estimated incidence of 43,700 new diagnoses (men = 23,400; women = 20,300) and an estimated 21,700 deaths (men = 11,500; women = 10,200). According to the International Agency for Research on Cancer, in 2000, there were 1,198,370 new diagnoses of cancer in Europe among people over 65 (52% of all malignant tumors) [4]. A total of 907,339 older adults died of cancer, accounting for 59% of all cancer deaths (EUROCARE 5 Study) [4]. In 2016, in Italy, just over 365,000 new cases were diagnosed, approximately 190,000 (54%) in men and 175,000 (46%) in women [4, 5]. The highest number of cancers are diagnosed among older adults (70+ years of age), accounting for over 50% of the total. Twenty percent of all cancers are diagnosed among those over 80, representing approximately two cases per 100 women and three to four cases per 100 men each year. According to the International Agency for Research on Cancer, in 2000, 1,198,370 new cases of cancer were diagnosed in Europe among people over 65, representing 52% of all malignant tumors [6].

In the past, many arguments were raised against the use of ERAS® protocols in older adults: lower compliance, the hypothesis that they might not tolerate early feeding after surgery, early enforced mobilization, and the perceived need for a longer convalescence after major surgery. On the contrary, many papers in the literature demonstrate beneficial effects of adopting fast-track protocols for colorectal surgery in older patients [6].

The ERAS® Society guidelines, revised in 2019 [7], cover many items and divide the protocol into five steps: preadmission, preoperative, intraoperative, postoperative, and discharge.

6.2 Preadmission

At preadmission, the first step is informing all parties involved, bearing in mind that patients are often affected by neurological disorders or sensory deficits (hearing, speech). That's why information about the protocol is important and should preferably be provided in the presence of younger relatives.

Moreover, assessing cognitive function is crucial to provide adequate education and counseling to patients and their families. Cognitive function is one of the items to be evaluated as part of the frailty assessment. Frailty can be understood in different ways: as the result of an accumulation of deficits (diseases, signs, symptoms, disabilities) that make the individual more vulnerable to complications, morbidity, and mortality or as a loss of homeostatic capacity, reduced resilience and adaptive ability of biological systems to environmental stressors. It is part of the aging process, distinct from disability and comorbidity, though closely interconnected.

Assessment of frailty is mandatory to identify how far our surgical action can be pushed. Determining a patient's preoperative frailty status is crucial for assessing perioperative risk, postoperative complications, increased length of hospital stay (LOS), increased mortality, higher level of care needed at discharge, and higher readmission rates [7].

Moreover, preoperative knowledge of frailty status can guide discussions among patients, their families, anesthesiologists, and surgeons to personalize perioperative, intraoperative, and postoperative care, including type of anesthesia and surgical procedure, in order to mitigate risk.

The Comprehensive Geriatric Assessment (CGA) is a multidisciplinary assessment that identifies, describes, and explains the multiple problems of older adults, catalogs their resources and strengths, assesses service needs, and develops a coordinated care plan.

An assessment with graduated scales or simple tests can identify a patient's weak points and initiate preoperative optimization. This phase is called prehabilitation and consists of correcting anemia and nutritional deficiencies, evaluating neurologic, cardiac, and respiratory disorders, improving global capacity, and optimizing overall function. This phase is extremely important for older patients and is now considered one of the essential items of the protocol, as reported in by Wang and colleagues [8]. Before surgery, patients should be brought to the best possible physical condition. The most fragile patients are recommended for a training program (physiotherapy, exercise, and sports therapy) to improve the musculoskeletal system, cardiovascular system, lung function, metabolism, and immune system.

The time between preoperative evaluation and surgery represents a valuable opportunity to increase functional reserves through optimizing medications, enhancing cognitive function, improving psychological state, planning structured exercises, and correcting nutritional deficiencies.

By adopting these pre-habilitation strategies, surgical outcomes can significantly improve, especially in frail patients. A meta-analysis [9] reported the effect of preoperative exercise and respiratory therapy on surgical outcomes in patients with lung cancer and chronic obstructive pulmonary disease (COPD): patients who received preoperative training showed a lower incidence of postoperative pulmonary complications and a shorter hospital stay. Patients with COPD did not experience fewer postoperative complications, but they did recover more quickly.

Nutritional support is a key aspect of perioperative management and is an increasingly integral part of many surgical programs. Malnutrition (sarcopenia) is very common in the elderly population and has a major clinical impact, particularly in patients with gastrointestinal malignancies, where the prevalence of malnutrition exceeds 38.5% [10]. The European Society for Clinical Nutrition and Metabolism (ESPEN) has established enteral nutrition guidelines for the postoperative phase in elderly patients. Perioperative nutritional support has been introduced in many consensus statements and guidelines [11]. In particular, adequate protein intake plays an important role, as it forms the basis for the supply of amino acids to the muscles. Preoperative nutritional status is a critical determinant of optimal outcomes for gastrointestinal cancer surgery; however, there is no consensus on how to accurately assess preoperative nutritional status. The European Society of Surgical Oncology and the ERAS® Society, in a position paper published in the European Journal of Surgical Oncology, proposed a Nutritional Risk Screening Score (NRS 2002) identifying eight key points [12]:

(a) integration of nutrition into overall patient management;
(b) avoidance of long periods of preoperative fasting;

(c) re-establishment of oral feeding as early as possible after surgery;
(d) early initiation of nutritional therapy as soon as nutritional risk becomes apparent;
(e) metabolic control (e.g., of blood glucose);
(f) reduction of factors that exacerbate stress-related catabolism or impair gastrointestinal function;
(g) early mobilization to facilitate protein synthesis and muscle function;
(h) minimizing time on paralytic agents for ventilator management in the postoperative period.

Forsmo and colleagues [13] conducted a study aiming to evaluate patients in different age groups within the ERAS® care pathway to determine whether elderly patients achieved the same outcomes as younger patients. Elderly patients' adherence to an ERAS® program was also compared with that of younger patients. Patients were divided into three groups based on age: ≤65 years (n = 79), 66–79 years (n = 56), and ≥ 80 years (n = 19). The primary endpoint was postoperative hospital stay (PHS) plus any additional days of readmission within the first 30 days after surgery. Secondary endpoints were postoperative complications, PHS, readmission rate, postoperative C-reactive protein (CRP) levels, mortality, and patient compliance with the different ERAS® elements. At the end of the study, there were no differences in morbidity or 30-day mortality. The lack of significant difference was attributed to logistical challenges, such as home care situation or the patient's own wishes.

We also have to consider polypharmacy, which is highly prevalent among older adults. Many patients take multiple medications, including anticoagulants, antiplatelets, antihypertensives, and psychotropics, all of which can increase the risk of perioperative complications. A structured medication review, ideally conducted in collaboration with a clinical pharmacist, can reduce the incidence of drug interactions and adverse events. Deprescribing unnecessary or harmful drugs in the weeks prior to surgery can enhance safety and improve functional recovery.

Furthermore, sensory impairment (hearing loss, reduced vision) may limit the ability of elderly patients to understand preoperative instructions. Providing written materials in large font, using visual aids, or involving caregivers ensures better comprehension and compliance. This highlights the importance of tailoring communication strategies to the specific vulnerabilities of geriatric patients.

6.3 Admission

Admission of the patient should be scheduled as close as possible to the operation and several aspects must be managed: optimize fluid hydration, avoid premedication and bowel preparation, obtain informed consent, and administer selected antibiotic prophylaxis for the scheduled surgery.

6.4 Intraoperative

Opiate-sparing analgesia, appropriate fluid management, and minimally invasive surgery are the three cornerstones of proper intraoperative management in the ERAS® protocol for colorectal surgery and beyond. Through epidural blockade or spinal anesthesia, the use of lidocaine in abdominal wall blocks, and laparoscopic transversus abdominis plane (TAP) blocks are the main standard procedures for anesthesia and management of postoperative analgesia.

In elderly patients, the use of bispectral index (BIS) monitoring to assess anesthesia depth is also very important. Adequate balance in fluid therapy, particularly the application of the concept of euvolemia (correcting any preoperative fluid or electrolyte excesses or deficits), is mandatory.

Arguments against using ERAS® in older adults are contradicted by the large number of papers in favor, present in the literature [14].

Surgeons will also try to avoid nasogastric tubes and remove urinary catheters and abdominal drains as soon as possible. The introduction of fast-track protocols in colorectal minimally invasive surgery (MIS) for the elderly produced an unexpected result: extremely good compliance and reduced postoperative morbidity. These two results translated into a significant reduction in LOS, greater than originally expected [15, 16]. Another intraoperative challenge in elderly patients is temperature control. Hypothermia during surgery is more common in older adults due to reduced thermoregulation and has been associated with increased risk of wound infections, coagulopathy, and delayed recovery from anesthesia. Active warming devices, warmed intravenous fluids, and careful monitoring of core temperature should therefore be considered integral components of the ERAS® pathway for this population. Equally important is the prevention of delirium, a frequent postoperative complication in the elderly. Intraoperative strategies such as minimizing the use of benzodiazepines, ensuring adequate pain control without excessive opioids, and maintaining hemodynamic stability can reduce its incidence. Delirium not only prolongs hospital stay but is also associated with long-term cognitive decline and increased mortality.

The role of MIS is well established, and MIS has become the standard of care (laparoscopic or robotic), fulfilling the intraoperative requirements of the ERAS® protocol. A minimally invasive approach has clear advantages: faster recovery, fewer general complications, fewer wound-related complications (including incisional hernia), and fewer adhesions [14–17].

Tejedor and colleagues [18] retrospectively analyzed 70,655 elderly patients who underwent colorectal surgery, divided into two groups: the first treated with laparoscopic surgery (LPS) and the second with laparotomic surgery (LPT). The proportion of LPT cases increased until 2013, then declined as open surgery decreased. All patients were included in a multivariate analysis, and the LPS group demonstrated lower mean total costs ($ 4012 less per case), fewer complications (−36%), and lower readmission rates (−33%) compared with the LPT group. Moreover, the LPS group had a shorter LOS (2.6 fewer days) than open cases and fewer severe complications. Considering readmission episodes, the MIS group proved less costly than the open group. Patients enrolled in an ERAS® protocol from 2018 to 2022 showed no significant differences in terms of sex, site, or surgical approach. However, in multivariate analysis, the elderly group demonstrated a significant reduction in morbidity (−69%; OR = 0.31; p = 0.030). No statistically significant difference was reported when applied to the entire population examined.

Wang et al. [8] analyzed 78 patients aged 65 or older who underwent laparoscopic colorectal resection for colorectal cancer between April 2006 and October 2009, divided into two groups: 40 patients treated under a fast-track protocol and 38 controls. The evaluation of recovery parameters showed statistically significant differences in favor of the ERAS® group for: time to first ambulation (p = 0.009), first flatus (p = 0.001), bowel movement (p = 0.001), time until diet (p = 0.001), and LOS (p = 0.001). No statistical differences were observed between the two groups for anastomotic leakage, pulmonary infection, or incision infection; a difference was found only in overall complications: 2 (5%) in the fast-track group vs. 8 (21.1%) in controls, p = 0.045.

6.5 Discharge

Post-discharge care is another crucial component. In this selected group of patients, fast-track protocols achieve goals more relevant to those obtained in younger patients. In fact, considering the beneficial effect of a shorter LOS in older patients, we more frequently obtain a return to their own home, maintenance of a good quality of life, and preservation of autonomy. Implementation of ERAS® pathways represents a significant advancement in optimizing discharge processes for elderly patients. By standardizing perioperative care through evidence-based interventions, ERAS® contributes to reducing postoperative complications, shortening hospital stays, and facilitating a timely yet safe discharge. When adapted to the specific vulnerabilities of the geriatric population, these protocols not only improve clinical outcomes but also support functional recovery and autonomy, thereby addressing both medical and social dimensions of care in the elderly. All authors agree that the presence of a multidisciplinary board, the evaluation of a CGA, and a dedicated multidisciplinary team—including geriatricians—are necessary to select the best clinical course and tailor surgery for frail patients. Elderly patients discharged early under ERAS® protocols require structured follow-up to prevent readmissions. Telephone check-ins, telemedicine consultations, and the involvement of community nurses have proven effective in monitoring recovery at home. Moreover, the presence of a caregiver or family support system strongly influences outcomes, underlining the need to integrate social resources into discharge planning. Several studies have demonstrated that when elderly patients are discharged under ERAS® protocols with adequate home support, rates of institutionalization in nursing homes are significantly reduced. This not only preserves autonomy and quality of life but also decreases the long-term burden on the healthcare system.

6.6 Conclusion

ERAS® represents a multidisciplinary approach consisting of a series of evidence-based perioperative interventions aimed at preserving immune function and enhancing recovery. Fast-track programs are now applied to many types of major surgery and are well known to reduce morbidity (by 50%), hospitalization (by 30%), and costs, while improving short-term outcomes and minimizing the surgical stress response caused by injury.

This new treatment "philosophy" is widely adopted in the elderly and has been slightly modified to improve compliance and outcomes in this selected population. LOS, return home, maintaining quality of life, avoiding loss of autonomy, and survival are key outcomes for elderly patients after surgery [19].

Many frail, elderly patients, who were sometimes excluded from ERAS® programs, can also benefit from a combination of a personalized prehabilitation program and ERAS® elements. In fact, adding a multimodal prehabilitation program at diagnosis to an ERAS® pathway before surgery may create complementary benefits and lead to functional improvements. Careful selection of frail patients is mandatory before making surgical decisions.

Colorectal surgery is one of the broadest fields in which the ERAS® "philosophy" has been tested in the literature. Research has revealed good protocol compliance and equivalent immediate and late results in terms of surgical site infection, postoperative stay, overall morbidity, and postoperative readmission rates, with minimal differences compared to younger patients.

A dedicated and integrated multidisciplinary team, including geriatricians, is essential. The multidisciplinary management of older surgical patients, integrating the expertise of surgeons, anesthetists, geriatricians, and other specialists and health care professionals, is necessary to continually improve short- and long-term outcomes in elderly patients undergoing colorectal surgery.

A relevant number of general statements can be made about the perioperative care of geriatric surgical patients, but ERAS® protocols are often "warmly" recommended in all older candidates for elective colorectal surgery [20]. In the near future, ERAS® protocols will likely evolve toward even greater personalization through the integration of digital health tools and artificial intelligence. Wearable devices capable of continuously monitoring vital parameters, mobility, and sleep patterns could provide real-time feedback on postoperative recovery, allowing the healthcare team to intervene promptly in the case of complications. Furthermore, predictive algorithms could stratify elderly patients according to individual risk, guiding the intensity of prehabilitation programs and tailoring perioperative interventions.

Ultimately, the ERAS® approach in the elderly should be seen not merely as a set of perioperative interventions but as a paradigm shift in the way surgical care is conceived: from a disease-centered model to a patient-centered, holistic, and multidisciplinary model.

References

1. Correra M. Boom di interventi chirurgici sugli anziani, 900mila l'anno [Internet]. National Associated Press Agency (ANSA); 2018 Jan [cited 2025 Sept 15]. Available from: https://www.ansa.it/canale_saluteebenessere/notizie/salute_65plus/medicina/2018/01/21/ansa-boom-di-interventi-chirurgici-sugli-anziani900mila-lanno_e78c168a-dce4-4487-a7d7-8759b4d9ce7a.html.
2. Bardram L, Funch-Jensen P, Jensen P, et al. Recovery after laparoscopic colonic surgery with epidural analgesia, and early oral nutrition and mobilisation. Lancet. 1995;345(8952):763–4.
3. Jia Y, Jin G, Guo S, et al. Fast-track surgery decreases the incidence of postoperative delirium and other complications in elderly patients with colorectal carcinoma. Langenbeck's Arch Surg. 2014;399(1):77–84.
4. AIOM – Associazione Italiana di Oncologia Medica. Linee guida tumori dell'anziano [Internet]. AIOM; 2018 [cited 2025 Sept 15]. Available from: https://www.sigg.it/wp-content/uploads/2019/02/2018_LG_AIOM_Tumori-Anziano.pdf.
5. Rossi S, Baili P, Capocaccia R, et al. The EUROCARE-5 study survival in Europe 1999-2007: database, quality on cancer checks and statistical analysis methods. Eur J Cancer. 2015;51(15):2104–19.
6. Bray F, Colombet M, Aitken JF, Bardot A, Eser S, Galceran J, et al., editors. Cancer incidence in five continents, Vol. XII. IARC Scientific Publication No. 169. Lyon: International Agency for Research on Cancer; 2024.
7. Gustafsson UO, Scott MJ, Hubner M, et al. Guidelines for perioperative care in elective colorectal surgery: enhanced recovery after surgery (ERAS®) society recommendations: 2018. World J Surg. 2019;43(3):659–95.
8. Wang Q, Suo J, Jiang J, et al. Effectiveness of fast-track rehabilitation vs conventional care in laparoscopic colorectal resection for elderly patients: a randomized trial. Color Dis. 2012;14(8):1009–13.
9. Wang L, Yu M, Ma Y, et al. Effect of pulmonary rehabilitation on postoperative clinical status in patients with lung cancer and chronic obstructive pulmonary disease: a systematic review and meta-analysis. Evid Based Complement Alternat Med. 2022;2022:4133237.
10. Ai D, Ding N, Wu H. The impact of sarcopenia on nutritional status in elderly patients with gastrointestinal tumors. Sci Rep. 2023;13(1):10308.
11. Weimann A, Braga M, Carli F, et al. ESPEN guideline: clinical nutrition in surgery. Clin Nutr. 2017;36(3):623–50.
12. Sandrucci S, Beets G, Braga M, et al. Perioperative nutrition and enhanced recovery after surgery in gastrointestinal cancer patients. A position paper by the ESSO task force in collaboration with the ERAS society (ERAS coalition). Eur J Surg Oncol. 2018;44(4):509–14.
13. Forsmo HM, Erichsen C, Rasdal A, et al. Enhanced recovery after colorectal surgery (ERAS) in elderly patients is feasible and achieves similar results as in younger patients. Gerontol Geriatr Med. 2017;3:2333721417706299.
14. Millan M, Renau-Escrig AI. Minimizing the impact of colorectal surgery in the older patient: the role of enhanced recovery programs in older patients. Eur J Surg Oncol. 2020;46(3):338–43.
15. Pache B, Hübner M, Jurt J, et al. Minimally invasive surgery and enhanced recovery after surgery: the ideal combination? J Surg Oncol. 2017;116(5):613–6.
16. Sood A, Meyer CP, Abdollah F, et al. Minimally invasive surgery and its impact on 30-day postoperative complications, unplanned readmissions and mortality. Br J Surg. 2017;104(10):1372–81.
17. Robinson CN, Balentine CJ, Marshall CL, et al. Minimally invasive surgery improves short-term outcomes in elderly colorectal cancer patients. J Surg Res. 2011;166(2):182–8.
18. Keller DS, Qiu J, Kiran RP. A national study on the adoption of laparoscopic colorectal surgery in the elderly population: current state and value proposition. Tech Coloproctol. 2019;23(10):965–72.

19. Gonzalez-Ayora S, Pastor C, Guadalajara H, et al. Enhanced recovery care after colorectal surgery in elderly patients. Compliance and outcomes of a multicenter study from the Spanish working group on ERAS. Int J Color Dis. 2016;31(9):1625–31.
20. Aceto P, Antonelli Incalzi R, Bettelli G, et al. Perioperative management of elderly patients (PriME): recommendations from an Italian intersociety consensus. Aging Clin Exp Res. 2020;32(9):1647–73.

Breast Surgery

7

Angela Gurrado, Lucia Ilaria Sgaramella, Francesco Paolo Prete, and Mario Testini

7.1 Epidemiology

Breast cancer (BC) is the leading cause of cancer morbidity, disability and mortality in women worldwide. In Europe the estimated incidence is 147.6 per 100,000 population, whereas in Italy 55,900 new diagnoses were estimated in 2023 [1–3].

Despite increasing incidence rates, mortality has gradually declined annually from 2011 to 2020, reaching its lowest levels at 1.3%, with a 5-year survival rate of 88% [4].

The main risk factors include age, reproductive factors, hormonal factors, dietary and metabolic factors, lifestyle, previous chest radiotherapy, history of breast dysplasia or neoplasia, family history, and hereditary predisposition. Among these, age is the most significant risk factor for BC.

The global increase in the aging population underscores the growing relevance of BC in elderly patients. In developed countries, up to 50% of BC diagnoses occur in women over the age of 65, and this proportion continues to rise [5–7].

According to data from the Italian Association of Tumor Registries (AIRTUM), in Italy 22% of new BC cases and 14% of BC-related deaths are expected to occur in women aged ≥70 years [2].

BC is also recognized as a common cause of death among older women. Among women aged ≥80 years at diagnosis, approximately 40% die because of the disease. Therefore, a thorough assessment of the patient's overall health status is essential [8].

These data highlight the importance of an appropriate diagnostic and therapeutic approach, particularly in elderly patients.

A. Gurrado (✉) · L. I. Sgaramella · F. P. Prete · M. Testini
Academic General Surgery Unit F. Paccione, Department of Precision and Regenerative Medicine and Jonian Area (DiMePRe-J), University of Bari Aldo Moro Medical School, Bari, Italy
e-mail: angela.gurrado@uniba.it; mario.testini@uniba.it

P. Carcoforo, F. Catena (eds.), *Geriatric Surgery*, Updates in Surgery,
https://doi.org/10.1007/978-3-032-24281-5_7

The International Society of Geriatric Oncology (SIOG) and the European Society of Breast Cancer Specialists (EUSOMA) recommend collaboration with geriatricians to optimize oncologic standards of care. They also advocate for the use of screening tools as a reasonable first step to identify patients who may benefit from a more comprehensive geriatric assessment [8].

7.2 Screening

It is true that there is a well-established diagnostic and therapeutic screening pathway for BC, but it is also evident that this pathway becomes less defined in older age groups. In fact, access to screening techniques in the elderly is often inconsistent and, in some cases, considered controversial.

Early screening techniques appear to reduce cancer-related mortality in elderly patients, except in those with limited life expectancy or severe comorbidities.

Current guidelines recommend biennial BC screening for all women starting at age 40 [8].

However, evidence remains inconclusive regarding the benefits and harms of continued screening beyond age 75, as well as the optimal screening strategies for women with dense breast tissue.

Several organizations, including the American Academy of Physicians, the American Academy of Family Physicians, and the U.S. Preventive Services Task Force, recommend discontinuing screening at age 74. The American Cancer Society recommends continuing BC screening in individuals with a life expectancy exceeding 10 years, whereas the American College of Physicians advises discontinuing screening by age 75 or earlier if life expectancy is less than 10 years [9].

This leads to an underrepresentation of patients over 75 years of age in screening programs and clinical studies, resulting in insufficient evidence to clearly determine whether BC screening should be continued or discontinued in this population.

Moreover, no randomized controlled trials have specifically assessed the efficacy of screening mammography in women aged 75 and older, and only a limited number of studies have included participants over 70 years of age, resulting in uncertainty regarding the benefits of screening and the risk of overdiagnosis within this population [9].

Overdiagnosis refers to the detection of a cancer through screening that would not have caused symptoms or harm during a person's lifetime. It is influenced by factors such as the tumor's biological behavior and the patient's life expectancy. Some BC have a long asymptomatic phase and may remain clinically silent if undetected, leading to potential overdiagnosis when found via screening [9].

The relative risk of overdiagnosis increases with age and is highest among the oldest women or those with the lowest life expectancy. Therefore, overdiagnosis should be explicitly considered alongside the potential benefits when making screening decisions. Decisions regarding the continuation of screening in this age group should be individualized, taking into account factors such as overall health status and prior screening history, while aiming to balance the benefits of cancer detection against the risks of overdiagnosis [10].

7.3 Biological Characteristics of Breast Cancer in Older Women

Older patients tend to present with biologically less aggressive BC, characterized by smaller tumor size, lower lymph node involvement, higher expression of estrogen and progesterone receptors, lower histologic grade, and more frequent human epidermal growth factor receptor (HER-2) negative status. These more favorable tumor phenotypes observed in older women are further supported by recent molecular genetic studies, which demonstrate an age-related increase in the prevalence of favorable BC subtypes, such as luminal A and luminal B. Although uncommon, unfavorable BC subtypes have been reported in older patients and are typically managed with more aggressive therapies [11].

A recent review analyzed the incidence of receptor status and corresponding molecular subtypes in BC among elderly patients. The findings showed that the incidence of luminal A subtypes ranged from 21.80% to 81.10%, luminal B from 7.10% to 33.30%, triple-negative subtypes from 8.90% to 20.30%, and HER2-enriched subtypes were reported in less than 16.10% of cases [12].

The small but significant increase in more favorable tumor characteristics and molecular subtypes observed in older patients has not translated into substantial improvements in survival, which may be partly explained by the fact that, in the absence of organized screening programs, diagnosis in older women often occurs at a more advanced stage of the disease [11, 13].

7.4 Indications for Surgical Treatment

A surgical approach remains a cornerstone in the management of BC; however, its implementation must be carefully balanced against tumor characteristics, patient-specific comorbidities, and individual preferences, while also considering the availability and appropriateness of alternative therapeutic options (radiation, chemotherapy, hormonal and endocrine therapy, adjuvant therapy, and neoadjuvant therapy).

The lack of a well-defined screening pathway for the elderly, combined with the exclusion of this population from prospective trials on tumor characterization, staging, and treatment, results in a significant gap in scientific evidence for patients over the age of 75. Therefore, treatment strategies for this age group are often suboptimal, being extrapolated from studies conducted on younger populations [12].

To address this gap, the most recent guidelines from the SIOG and the EUSOMA emphasize the need to consider breast-conserving surgery (BCS) followed by whole-breast radiotherapy, or mastectomy followed by postoperative radiotherapy in selected patients, as the standard of care for elderly patients with BC.

Indeed, recent literature shows that surgery is the primary method of treating BC, in most studies with favorable outcomes reporting an overall survival (OS) at 7 years of 95.2% and a disease-free survival (DFS) at 5 years of 84.6%.

The risk of postoperative complications increases with age; however, these events are generally mild to moderate in severity and are not associated with an increased risk of mortality. Moreover, inadequate local disease control can negatively impact both quality of life and functional status.

A systematic review of seven clinical trials (Cochrane Review; 1571 women, 12-year follow-up) evaluated primary endocrine therapy with tamoxifen alone versus surgery (with or without tamoxifen) in women aged ≥70 years with operable breast cancer who were fit for surgery [14].

The review reported the following key findings: no difference in OS was observed between treatment arms (1081 deaths among 1571 patients). The hazard ratio (HR) for OS was 0.98 for surgery versus primary endocrine therapy, and 0.86 for surgery plus adjuvant endocrine therapy versus primary endocrine therapy. A statistically significant improvement in progression-free survival was found in favor of surgery (with or without endocrine therapy). The HR for progression-free survival was 0.55 for surgery versus primary endocrine therapy, and 0.65 for surgery plus adjuvant endocrine therapy versus primary endocrine therapy.

Additionally, data from a large cohort study showed no significant difference in BC-specific survival between primary endocrine therapy and surgery in patients with early-stage, luminal A tumors.

When an aromatase inhibitor is used as primary endocrine therapy, the median time to progression is approximately 5 years. Therefore, the expected benefit from exclusive primary endocrine therapy is greater in women with a life expectancy of less than 5 years [15].

Therefore, despite the absence of a demonstrated OS benefit, surgery remains the standard of care due to its advantage in progression-free survival. Alternative therapeutic approaches should be considered only for patients with severe comorbidities that place them at high risk of death from competing non-cancer-related causes [8].

7.5 Axillary Management in Older Breast Cancer Patients

There is a growing global trend toward de-escalation of axillary surgery in older BC patients. Patient age, indeed, has become an integrated factor in the diagnostic and treatment algorithm for BC since the Milan III trial demonstrated that older women exhibited low rates of local recurrence, regardless of the administration of postoperative radiotherapy [16].

This approach is supported by an improved understanding of tumor biology, which is often more favorable in the geriatric population (HR+/HER2−, grade 1–2), and by the observation that approximately 70% of women over the age of 70 present with node-negative disease. Preoperative axillary ultrasound has proven to be a reliable tool for assessing nodal status in clinically node-negative (cN0) patients, with a sensitivity of approximately 80%. Its use may allow accurate staging potentially avoiding axillary surgery in selected cases, thereby reducing the risk of postoperative complications, which can significantly impact morbidity, particularly in frail elderly women. Omission of axillary staging compared to axillary lymph node dissection in elderly women with clinically node-negative axilla does not appear to have a negative impact on survival and is associated with a low incidence of local recurrence.

As part of the "Choosing Wisely Campaign", the Society of Surgical Oncology (SSO) has listed as its top recommendation the option to omit sentinel lymph node biopsy (SLNB) in clinically node-negative women over the age of 70 with hormone receptor-positive, ERBB2-negative tumors. The SSO emphasizes that axillary staging should be considered on an individual basis, particularly when the results are likely to influence decisions regarding adjuvant systemic therapy or locoregional radiotherapy [8].

Nevertheless, as previously noted in the context of ductal carcinoma *in situ*, the use of SLNB in elderly patients remains high, despite growing evidence supporting its de-escalation. Population-based datasets and single-institution studies report SLNB rates ranging from 80% to 88% in women over 70, and between 46% and 76% in those over 80 years of age [16].

While SLNB remains appropriate in selected cases where treatment decisions depend on nodal status, the increasing adoption of genomic assays to guide systemic therapy, along with the low incidence of axillary recurrence in older women, suggests that omission of SLNB should be considered in elderly patients with biologically favorable tumors.

7.6 Postoperative Radiotherapy in Older Breast Cancer Patients

As with axillary surgery, there is a global trend toward de-escalation in the use of postoperative radiotherapy in BC treatment. Several studies have already explored this approach.

In a landmark study with long-term follow-up, Hughes KS et al. analyzed 636 women aged ≥70 years with hormone receptor-positive, clinical stage I breast cancer (cT1, cN0) who underwent BCS and were then randomized to receive either tamoxifen alone or whole-breast irradiation (WBI) plus tamoxifen. At a median follow-up of 12.6 years, the study demonstrated no significant differences between the two groups in terms of OS, distant metastasis-free survival, incidence of second primary tumors, or mastectomy rates (including those performed after recurrence). The only significant difference observed was in locoregional recurrence rates: at 10 years, 90% of patients treated with tamoxifen alone (95% CI, 85–93%) remained free of locoregional recurrence, compared to 98% of those who also received radiotherapy (95% CI, 96–99%) [17, 18].

In the PRIME II trial, 1326 women aged ≥65 years with hormone receptor-positive BC measuring up to 3 cm, node-negative (N0), with clear surgical margins (R0), and receiving adjuvant endocrine therapy were randomized to receive or omit adjuvant radiotherapy. At a median follow-up of 5 years, the primary endpoint—ipsilateral breast tumor recurrence—was 1.3% in the radiotherapy group and 4.1% in the no-radiotherapy group (HR 5.19; p = 0.0002). No significant differences were observed between the two groups in terms of regional recurrences, distant metastases, contralateral BC, or overall survival.

An updated analysis presented at SABCS 2020 confirmed a significantly higher rate of local recurrence at 10 years in patients who did not receive radiotherapy (9.8% vs. 0.9%) while the incidence of distant metastases, contralateral recurrences, and OS remained similar between groups [8, 19].

Furthermore, the St. Gallen 2021 consensus panel recommended the use of radiotherapy in older women with an estimated life expectancy exceeding 10 years, particularly in cases of tumors larger than 2.5 cm, lymph node involvement, or the presence of adverse biomolecular features [20].

The National Comprehensive Cancer Network (NCCN) guidelines consider that omission of radiotherapy may be proposed in patients aged 70 years or older with stage I, estrogen receptor-positive breast cancer who undergo BCS with negative margins and are receiving adjuvant endocrine therapy [21].

It is therefore reasonable to consider the omission of radiotherapy after surgery as a treatment option for highly selected patients with a life expectancy exceeding 10 years, following thorough multidisciplinary evaluation. In fact, it is recommended that in women aged ≥70 years who have undergone BCS for low-risk invasive BC and are receiving adjuvant endocrine therapy, the omission of WBI may be considered a valid alternative. In all cases, it is essential to provide patients with comprehensive information regarding the goals and expectations of treatment, to support the most personalized and informed decision-making process [8].

7.7 Adjuvant Systemic Therapy

The decision to offer adjuvant treatment to an elderly patient should be based on a careful balance between life expectancy and the risk of cancer recurrence. Currently, omission of adjuvant endocrine therapy may be considered an option in elderly women with a low-risk tumor—for example, pT1a G1—or in those with severe comorbidities.

In women diagnosed with operable, hormone receptor-positive (ER-positive and/or PgR-positive) invasive BC, the benefit of adjuvant endocrine therapy—either with tamoxifen or an aromatase inhibitor—is independent of age.Therefore, in elderly patients who are considered candidates for adjuvant hormonal treatment, it is appropriate to follow the same approach used in younger postmenopausal women. In the absence of absolute contraindications, an aromatase inhibitor should be considered as part of the adjuvant endocrine strategy, either in a sequential approach or as initial (upfront) therapy. Aromatase inhibitors are generally preferred over tamoxifen in elderly patients, as tamoxifen-related adverse effects are age-dependent; specifically, the risk of death from pulmonary embolism and endometrial cancer increases with advancing age. Nevertheless, the negative impact of aromatase inhibitors on bone density is particularly problematic in the elderly, where bone demineralization and osteoporosis are prevalent [8].

Recent studies have shown that in cases of HR+/HER2- BC in patients over 70 years of age, the addition of adjuvant chemotherapy to endocrine therapy is associated with improved survival outcomes while in cases of hormone receptor-negative or triple-negative tumors, adjuvant chemotherapy alone has demonstrated, however, survival benefits [8].

In fit elderly patients with operated BC who are candidates for adjuvant chemotherapy, a polychemotherapy regimen is recommended over monochemotherapy.

Regarding the choice of chemotherapy regimen, CMF (cyclophosphamide + methotrexate +5-fluorouracil), AC (doxorubicin + cyclophosphamide), and TC (docetaxel + cyclophosphamide) are regimens whose feasibility has been demonstrated in older women. The use of sequential regimens (e.g., anthracyclines followed by taxanes) in elderly patients is not supported by clinical trials. Therefore, such regimens should be reserved for "fit" patients with biologically aggressive tumors.

In older patients with biologically aggressive and/or advanced-stage BC who are not candidates for polychemotherapy due to poor general condition or high risk of toxicity, a personalized treatment approach may be considered. Although monochemotherapy with paclitaxel failed to demonstrate non-inferiority compared to the AC combination, its favorable toxicity profile and an absolute difference of only 1% in OS make paclitaxel a reasonable option for unfit patients who "require" chemotherapy

Moreover, in the "fit" elderly patient with operable HER2-positive BC larger than 1 cm or node-positive, the use of trastuzumab in combination with chemotherapy should be considered compared to chemotherapy alone.

Regarding the use of adjuvant trastuzumab, a consistent 3-year DFS rate was observed across different age groups starting from 40 years. In elderly patients receiving trastuzumab in combination with chemotherapy, there was a 47% reduction in the risk of recurrence compared to chemotherapy alone. However, the toxicity of chemotherapy regimens containing trastuzumab should be taken into consideration, as they are associated with a higher risk of adverse cardiac events in adult patients and a careful cost–benefit analysis of adjuvant treatment should be considered in elderly patients with low-risk HER2-positive tumors (i.e., T < 1 cm). Indeed, advanced age (>80 years), the presence of coronary artery disease and hypertension, as well as weekly administration of trastuzumab, are considered the main risk factors for a cardiac event.

The SIOG recommends the use of adjuvant chemotherapy in combination with one year of trastuzumab as the standard of care for elderly patients without cardiac dysfunction and with HER2-positive breast cancer of pT >0.5 cm, with escalation to dual HER2 blockade including trastuzumab in a limited subset of fit, high-risk patients.

References

1. Minhas A. Breast cancer incidence in women in European countries in 2022 [Internet]. 2025 [cited 2025 Aug 7]. Available from: https://www.statista.com/statistics/456804/breast-cancer-incidence-in-women-in-europe/?srsltid=AfmBOorCETKkJV7n7lhUkIfrfiLZvG6fE7DJp-GiU0SFuAoTIIGQkxoq.
2. I numeri del cancro in Italia 2023 [cited 2025 Aug 7]. Available from: https://www.aiom.it/wp-content/uploads/2024/02/2023_AIOM_NDC-web_def.pdf.
3. Bray F, Laversanne M, Sung H, et al. Global cancer statistics 2022: GLOBOCAN estimates of incidence and mortality worldwide for 36 cancers in 185 countries. CA Cancer J Clin. 2024;74(3):229–63.
4. Joseph K, Zebak S, Alba V, et al. Adjuvant breast radiotherapy, endocrine therapy, or both after breast conserving surgery in older women with low-risk breast cancer: results from a population-based study. Radiother Oncol. 2021;154:93–100.
5. Wildiers H, Kunkler I, Biganzoli L, et al. Management of breast cancer in elderly individuals: recommendations of the International Society of Geriatric Oncology. Lancet Oncol. 2007;8(12):1101–15.
6. Muss HB. Coming of age: breast cancer in seniors. Oncologist. 2011;16(Suppl 5):79–87.
7. Jemal A, Ward E, Thun MJ. Recent trends in breast cancer incidence rates by age and tumor characteristics among U.S. women. Breast Cancer Res. 2007;9(3):R28.
8. AIOM Linee guida del carcinoma mammario in stadio precoce [Internet]. AIOM; 2023 [cited 2025 Aug 19]. Available from: https://www.aiom.it/linee-guida-aiom-2023-carcinoma-mammario-in-stadio-precoce/.
9. Richman IB, Long JB, Soulos PR, et al. Estimating breast cancer overdiagnosis after screening mammography among older women in the United States. Ann Intern Med. 2023;176(9):1172–80.
10. US Preventive Services Task Force, Nicholson WK, Silverstein M, et al. Screening for breast cancer: US Preventive Services Task Force recommendation statement. JAMA. 2024;331(22):1918–30.
11. Karuturi M, VanderWalde N, Muss H. Approach and management of breast cancer in the elderly. Clin Geriatr Med. 2016;32(1):133–53.
12. Fonseca VC, Sidiropoulou Z. Geriatric breast cancer: staging, molecular surrogates, and treatment. A review & meta-analysis. Aging Dis. 2024;15(4):1602–18.
13. Gal O, Ishai Y, Sulkes A, et al. Early breast cancer in the elderly: characteristics, therapy, and long-term outcome. Oncology. 2018;94(1):31–8.
14. Hind D, Wyld L, Beverley CB, Reed MW. Surgery versus primary endocrine therapy for operable primary breast cancer in elderly women (70 years plus). Cochrane Database Syst Rev. 2006;1:CD004272.
15. Williams LJ, Kunkler IH, King CC, et al. A randomised controlled trial of post-operative radiotherapy following breast-conserving surgery in a minimum-risk population. Quality of life at 5 years in the PRIME trial. Health Technol Assess. 2011;15(12):i–xi, 1–57.
16. Hersh EH, King TA. De-escalating axillary surgery in early-stage breast cancer. Breast. 2022;62(Suppl 1):S43–9.
17. Hughes KS, Schnaper LA, Berry D, et al. Lumpectomy plus tamoxifen with or without irradiation in women 70 years of age or older with early breast cancer. N Engl J Med. 2024;351(10):971–7.
18. Hughes KS, Schnaper LA, Bellon JR, et al. Lumpectomy plus tamoxifen with or without irradiation in women age 70 years or older with early breast cancer: long-term follow-up of CALGB 9343. J Clin Oncol. 2013;31(19):2382–7.
19. Kunkler IH, Williams LJ, Jack WJL, et al. Breast-conserving surgery with or without irradiation in women aged 65 years or older with early breast cancer (PRIME II): a randomised controlled trial. Lancet Oncol. 2015;16:266–73.

20. Burstein HJ, Curigliano G, Thürlimann B, et al. Customizing local and systemic therapies for women with early breast cancer: the St. Gallen International Consensus Guidelines for treatment of early breast cancer 2021. Ann Oncol. 2021;32(10):1216–35.
21. Gradishar WJ, Moran MS, Abraham J, et al. Breast cancer, version 3.2024, NCCN clinical practice guidelines in oncology. J Natl Compr Cancer Netw. 2024;22(5):331–57.

Thyroid and Parathyroid Surgery in the Elderly

8

Giovanni Docimo, Eduardo Marcelo Iervolino, Maria Vittoria Zanzi, Eleonora Rossin, Giovanni Cozzolino, and Paolo Carcoforo

Among the various definitions of "elderly patients" in use, we believe Grogan's definition to be more comprehensive and better correlated with clinical data; patients aged 16 to 64 are classified as "young", those aged 65 to 79 as "elderly" and those aged 80 and over as "super-elderly" [1]. Current data from the Italian Statistics Institute (ISTAT) show that in Italy, the population aged over 65 will increase from 23.5% today to 34.9% by 2050 [2].

Thyroid nodules are an extremely common clinical condition in the general population, with an inevitable increase related to patient age. Older people show a higher prevalence of thyroid cancer in conjunction with increased comorbidities and functional decline. The absolute number of postoperative complications must be assessed in relation to coexisting comorbidities.

As aging of the population leads to a higher incidence of thyroid tumors, knowledge of the risks and benefits of thyroid surgery is a crucial point in the therapeutic pathway [3, 4].

The main indications for thyroid surgery in geriatric patients are:

- Suspected malignancy
- Thyrotoxicosis
- Compressive goiter.

G. Docimo · E. M. Iervolino · G. Cozzolino (✉)
Thyroid Surgery Unit, University of Campania Luigi Vanvitelli, Naples, Italy
e-mail: giovanni.docimo@unicampania.it; eduardomarcelo.iervolino@policliniconapoli.it; giovanni91cozzolino@libero.it

M. V. Zanzi · E. Rossin
Second Surgery Unit, Ferrara University Hospital, Ferrara, Italy
e-mail: znzmvt@unife.it; eleonora.rossin@ospfe.it

P. Carcoforo
Breast Surgery Unit, Ferrara University Hospital, Cona, Ferrara, Italy
e-mail: ccf@unife.it

P. Carcoforo, F. Catena (eds.), *Geriatric Surgery*, Updates in Surgery,
https://doi.org/10.1007/978-3-032-24281-5_8

Respiratory difficulties and dyspnea require preoperative cardiological and/or pulmonological diagnostic investigation.

The indications listed are shared by a large number of studies in the literature [5–7] (Table 8.1).

Although the oncological risk of thyroid nodules increases with age, the long-term negative effects of hyperfunctioning nodules (arrhythmias, osteoporosis, etc.) are not negligible.

While the progression of thyroid cancer in elderly patients is considered serious owing to a documented greater disease aggressiveness, the indications related to compressive pathology may be accompanied by numerous comorbidities linked to prolonged therapy undertaken in an attempt to avoid surgery.

Drug treatment with levothyroxine (LT4) has not only failed to demonstrate clinical improvements in halting nodular growth or reducing compressive symptoms, but has often proved disadvantageous, leading to the development of cardiovascular complications and severe osteoporosis with an increased risk of fractures, predominantly in female patients [8, 9].

Although in some published studies the indications for thyroid and parathyroid surgery in the elderly were approached with caution and established only in cases of actual necessity [10], the most recent data show the importance of distinguishing between chronological age and biological age, with the real determining factor being the coexistence of serious comorbidities at the time of surgery and not mere chronological age.

Based on the available literature data, the most common comorbidities in elderly patients are:

- Arterial hypertension
- Diabetes mellitus
- Ischemic heart disease
- Cardiac arrhythmias

Table 8.1 Baseline characteristics and indication for surgery. From [7] with permission

Variable	18–64 yrs (young)	65–74 yrs (older)	≥75 yrs (elderly)	*p*
Patients, n (%)	1499 (73.8)	370 (18.2)	161 (7.9)	–
Female sex, n (%)	1208 (80.6)	278 (75.1)	113 (70.2)	0.002
Family history, n (%)	765 (51.0)	152 (41.1)	51 (31.7)	<0.001
ASA I–II/III–IV, n (%)	1424 (95.0) / 75 (5.0)	290 (78.4) / 80 (21.6)	90 (55.9) / 71 (44.1)	<0.001
Abnormal laryngoscopy, n (%)	13 (0.9)	7 (1.9)	6 (3.7)	0.007
Indication for surgery				<0.001
Multinodular goiter, n (%)	715 (47.7)	239 (64.6)	113 (70.2)	
Graves' disease, n (%)	301 (20.1)	28 (7.6)	5 (3.1)	
Solitary nodule, n (%)	404 (27.0)	79 (21.4)	24 (14.9)	
Carcinoma, n (%)	60 (4.0)	14 (3.8)	10 (6.2)	
Other indications, n (%)	60 (4.0)	12 (3.2)	11 (6.9)	
Bethesda (I–V/not performed), n (%)	866 (57.7) / 605 (40.4)	194 (52.4) / 183 (49.5)	67 (41.6) / 88 (54.7)	0.001

- Lung diseases
- Neurological disorders.

In this regard, careful individual preoperative assessment is necessary in geriatric patients [11].

Based on data from most reviews in scientific literature, no substantial differences in the onset of postoperative complications are observed between "young" and "elderly" patients with the same American Society of Anesthesiologists (ASA) I-II classification [12].

The most common complications include (Table 8.2):

- Temporary/permanent hypocalcemia
- Temporary/permanent functional deficit of the recurrent laryngeal nerve (RLN)
- Hemorrhage
- Infections and hematomas of the wound.

Although in a clear minority, some authors (Passler et al.) previously emphasized the increased risk of reoperation, up to 38% in cases of submerged goiter in elderly patients [13].

Compressive goiter remains one of the main indications for surgery, without, however, neglecting the oncological data in elderly patients. Age plays a fundamental role in the progression of nodular pathology towards malignancy; this aspect is a prognostic factor that inevitably influences the outcome.

Furthermore, according to some studies, differentiated thyroid tumors (DTC) show greater aggressiveness correlated with more marked resistance to radioiodine therapy (RIT) in elderly patients and evidence of lymph node metastasis [14].

Table 8.2 Surgical morbidity. From [7] with permission

Outcome	18–64 yrs (young)	65–74 yrs (older)	≥75 yrs (elderly)	*p*
Reintervention for bleeding, n (%)	21 (1.4)	17 (4.6)	4 (2.5)	<0.001
Hypocalcemia (any), n (%)	244 (25.9)	61 (22.9)	35 (28.7)	0.425
Transient/permanent, n (%)	201 (21.3) / 43 (4.6)	44 (16.5) / 17 (6.4)	28 (23.0) / 7 (5.7)	0.428/—
RLN palsy (any), n (%)	67 (2.7)	23 (3.6)	13 (4.6)	0.147
Transient/permanent, n (%)	33 (1.4) / 34 (1.4)	10 (1.6) / 13 (2.1)	5 (1.8) / 8 (2.8)	0.417/—
LOS > 1 day, n (%)	147 (9.8)	75 (20.3)	70 (43.5)	<0.001
Wound morbidity, n (%)	37 (2.5)[a]	20 (5.4)[b]	7 (4.3)[c]	0.010
Clavien–Dindo ≥ 2, n (%)	82 (5.5)	33 (8.4)	21 (12.5)	<0.001
30-day mortality, n (%)	1 (0.1)	2 (0.5)	2 (1.2)	0.014
Calcium at 6 weeks, mmol/L, median (IQR)	2.36 (2.29–2.43)	2.36 (2.29–2.45)	2.34 (2.24–2.43)	0.166

[a]Fifteen seromas, twelve hematomas, three subcutaneous emphysema, two wound infections, two abscesses, two keloid formations, one wound dehiscence; [b]Nine hematomas, nine seromas and two wound infections; [c]Three hematomas, three seromas, one abscess; *IQR* interquartile range, *LOS* length of hospital stay, *RLN* recurrent laryngeal nerve

The mechanism underlying RIT resistance (radioactive iodine-refractory disease) is mainly linked to the lower expression of Na^{+} ion membrane transporters ("symporters"), which would limit the uptake of radioactive iodine. In addition, the main causes of increased aggressiveness include the activation of mitogen-activated protein kinases (MAPKs), which have a positive effect on the mitosis of endothelial cells and angiogenesis and increase the production of vascular endothelial and platelet-derived growth factors (VEGF, PDGF) [15].

Some authors have highlighted how the patient's age is associated with a higher incidence of papillary carcinoma specifically, without showing any particular variations for non-papillary carcinomas [16].

Nonetheless, scientific data agree in correlating the success of surgical treatment above all to the coexistence of comorbidities prior to surgery, independent of thyroid or parathyroid disease [17–19].

Today, there are a number of tools available to assist in assessing preoperative risk, such as the Surgical Risk Calculator provided by the website of the American College of Surgeons [11].

Online risk calculators are tables that can be filled in online. They calculate preoperative risk based on clinical and biological parameters, providing surgeons with a valuable tool for therapeutic assessment [20] (Fig. 8.1).

The assessment of the patient's frailty must not only take into account their clinical condition and biological parameters, but also the psychological aspects that inevitably affect their ability to cope with peri- and postoperative stress, as well as those related to everyday life [21].

There is no shortage of scientific studies highlighting that elderly patients more frequently require to be readmitted and have longer hospital stays (43.5% for

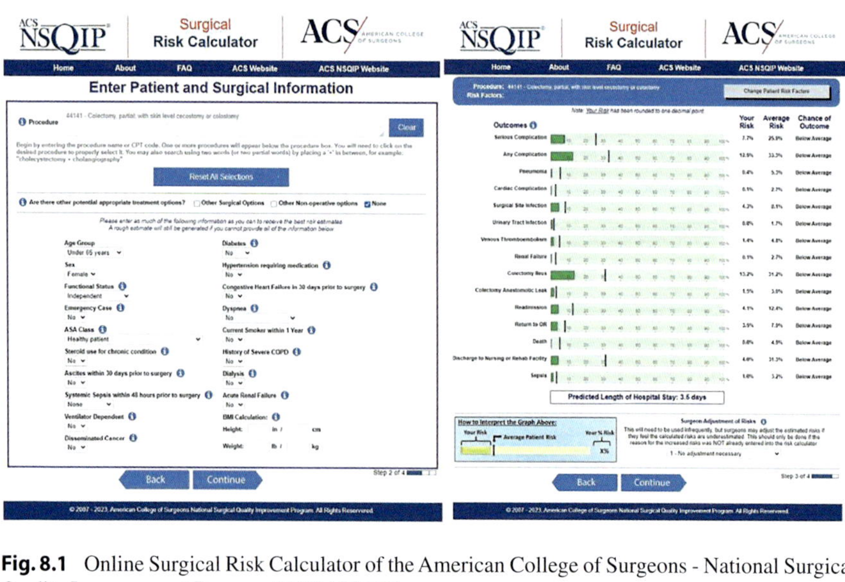

Fig. 8.1 Online Surgical Risk Calculator of the American College of Surgeons - National Surgical Quality Improvement Program (ACS-NSQIP)

patients >75 years of age vs. 9.8% <64 years), with an inevitable increase in health-care costs (4.6% for the 65–74 age group and 2.5% for those aged over 75 years vs. 1.4% <64 years of age). However, complications directly related to surgery, such as hypocalcemia and RLN paralysis, do not show substantial variations compared to younger patients [7].

8.1 Anaplastic Carcinomas

Although less common (2–3% of all thyroid neoplasms), it is worth mentioning anaplastic carcinomas. They typically occur in patients with an average age of 65, more commonly in women, and can be considered systemic diseases in light of their rapid local spread and high percentage of distant metastases, already present at diagnosis (50%), and local infiltration. Twenty per cent of patients with anaplastic thyroid carcinoma have a clinical history of concomitant differentiated thyroid carcinoma or chronic multinodular goiter; sometimes anaplastic carcinomas represent the evolution of some DTCs. For this reason, the molecular pathogenesis appears to be similar to that of DTCs (*BRAF*, *NTRK*, *RET*, *ALK* genes). Although the average survival rate is very low (4–6 months from diagnosis), it appears to have improved for *BRAF*-mutated patients treated with recently introduced targeted therapies (dabrafenib/trametinib) [22, 23].

8.2 Medullary Carcinomas

Medullary carcinomas account for approximately 5% of thyroid tumors, and their incidence is increasing [24].

The 10-year survival rate is approximately 65–71%, with a rate of distant metastasis of approximately 40–44%. However, the correlation between the increase and age in disease-specific mortality is controversial in the literature. A combination of factors, including the increased percentage of elderly patients (aged ≥65 years), the increased incidence of thyroid cancer and, not least, advances in surgical techniques have made it possible to increase the number of surgical procedures for geriatric patients over the years. Even for these tumors, elderly patients tend to present at advanced stages of the disease and with a more aggressive histology. The absolute data highlighted by a recent study show that, out of 1457 patients, medullary carcinoma-specific mortality was 2.9 and 6.7 times more likely for patients aged 65–79 and >80 years, respectively [25].

However, the scientific community is almost unanimous in confirming that the patient's age alone cannot be considered an absolute contraindication to surgical treatment.

8.3 Ablative Methods

Although ablative methods (radiofrequency, laser, microwave, and alcohol ablation for colloid-cystic nodules) were developed for the treatment of benign thyroid nodules, from the outset they were indicated in the literature as palliative treatments in cancer patients who were inoperable or refractory to radioiodine therapy [26]. Alcohol ablation is now exclusively indicated for the treatment of benign colloid-cystic lesions.

Most authors also assume the possibility of treating microcarcinomas with thermoablation methods, but the debate on this issue is still open and heated.

The main indications for thermoablation treatment in elderly patients with benign nodules include cosmetic problems, pain, dysphagia, foreign body sensation, discomfort, cough, cervical obstruction, and tracheal compression. The complex anatomy of the neck involves the onset of certain complications, albeit to a lesser extent than with surgical methods. In radiofrequency thermal ablation, damage to the RLN is more common, with rates of approximately 0.9% (vs. 0.4–7.2% for surgical thyroidectomies) for temporary lesions and 0.04% (vs. 0–5.2%) for permanent lesions [27]. The same author highlights a low incidence of hypothyroidism compared to surgical patients (0.04%).

According to the literature, when comparing the various thermoablation methods evaluated in the treatment of benign nodules, all methods showed a consistent reduction in nodule volume over time in elderly patients, with a slight advantage in favor of laser ablation, mainly evident in the first 6 months after treatment [28].

According to the guidelines, thermal ablation methods can be considered valid alternatives to surgical treatment in patients over 65, offering a good safety profile for the patient and a minimal incidence of postoperative complications.

8.4 Parathyroidectomy in Elderly Patients

Primary hyperparathyroidism (PHPT) is a condition responsible for numerous possible clinical implications; among these, the reduction in bone mineral density values is of great importance.

PHPT can be defined as a pathological condition in which blood PTH levels are elevated or "inadequately normal", resulting in elevated blood Ca^{++} levels. PHPT is often diagnosed late due to its subtle symptoms, which are often masked by comorbidities associated with the patient's advanced age in the early stages of the disease, becoming apparent only after damage has occurred.

Parathyroidectomy surgery remains the only truly effective treatment for this condition. The most important indications include:

- Osteoporosis
- Radiographic evidence of vertebral fragility/collapse.

The coexistence of osteoporosis in HPT is reported to have an increased incidence ranging between 39–63% [29–31]. A fact that should not be underestimated is that elderly patients not only have a generally increased risk of bone fractures, but that pelvic fractures in particular are associated with an increase in mortality between 18.6% and 24.5% in the following year [31].

The most common surgical complications observed in elderly patients are:

- Wound hematomas
- Seromas
- Cardiopulmonary complications
- Hypocalcemia (<7.5 mg/dL) with readmission within 30 days
- Permanent hypocalcemia (>6 months after surgery)
- Iatrogenic RLN lesions.

Most studies in the literature show that the postoperative complications of parathyroidectomy in HPT are comparable in patients ≤75 years of age compared to those ≤65 years of age, in the absence of serious comorbidities, comparable to those considered for elective inguinal hernia surgery [32]. This data would confirm parathyroidectomy as a safe procedure for elderly patients.

In the 6 months following surgery, there was an improvement in bone density, accompanied by a reduced percentage of fractures due to bone fragility. This benefit appears to be more evident in patients aged ≤75 years than in patients >75 years, emphasizing that in cases of HPT, it is better for those over 65 to undergo surgery at an early stage [29]. The same source also reports that cardiopulmonary complications gradually increase after the age of 75.

In conclusion, parathyroidectomy can be defined as a safe surgical procedure in the elderly, as can total thyroidectomy, since advanced age cannot be considered an absolute contraindication to surgery [33].

References

1. Grogan RH, Mitmaker EJ, Hwang J, et al. A population-based prospective cohort study of complications after thyroidectomy in the elderly. J Clin Endocrinol Metab. 2012;97(5):1645–53.
2. Istat. Le condizioni di salute della popolazione anziana in Italia. Anno 2019 [Internet]. Istat 2021 Jul [cited 2025 Sept 15]. Available from: https://www.istat.it/it/files/2021/07/Report-anziani-2019.pdf.
3. Ospina NS, Papaleontiou M. Thyroid nodule evaluation and management in older adults: a review of practical considerations for clinical endocrinologists. Endocr Pract. 2021;27(3):261–8.
4. Lim H, Devesa SS, Sosa JA, et al. Trends in thyroid cancer incidence and mortality in the United States, 1974-2013. JAMA. 2017;317(13):1338–48.
5. Ataş H, Nasıroğlu İmga N. Comparative outcomes of thyroid surgery in elderly patients: a retrospective cohort study. J Surg Med. 2020;4(10):879–82.
6. Tartaglia F, Russo G, Sgueglia M, et al. Total thyroidectomy in geriatric patients: a retrospective study. Int J Surg. 2014;12(Suppl 2):S33–6.
7. Van den Eynde F, Van Den Heede K, Brusselaers N, Van Slycke S. Thyroid surgery in the elderly: a surgical cohort. Langenbeck's Arch Surg. 2023;408(1):254.

8. Gluvic Z, Obradovic M, Stewart AJ, et al. Levothyroxine treatment and the risk of cardiac arrhythmias - focus on the patient submitted to thyroid surgery. Front Endocrinol (Lausanne). 2021;12:758043.
9. Chen CY, Chen ST, Huang BY, et al. The effect of suppressive thyroxine therapy in nodular goiter in postmenopausal women and 2 year's bone mineral density change. Endocr J. 2018;65(11):1101–9.
10. Sakowitz S, Bakhtiyar SS, Khoraminejad B, et al. Thyroid surgery outcomes in octogenarians: a national analysis. Surgery. 2023;174(1):52–8.
11. McIntire JB, McCammon S, Mong ER. Endocrine surgery in the geriatric population. Otolaryngol Clin N Am. 2018;51(4):753–8.
12. Chong MJ, Chooi JE. Commentary on: risk factors for postoperative morbidity after thyroid surgery in a PROSPECTIVE cohort of 1500 patients (Int. J. Surg. 2021, Epub ahead of print). Int J Surg. 2021;90:105975.
13. Passler C, Avanessian R, Kaczirek K, et al. Thyroid surgery in the geriatric patient. Arch Surg. 2002;137(11):1243–8.
14. Zhang Y, Ji X, Yang Z, Wang Y. Risk factors for cervical lymph node metastasis of papillary thyroid cancer in elderly patients aged 65 and older. Front Endocrinol (Lausanne). 2024;15:1418767.
15. Gosain R, Alexander JS, Gill A, Perez C. Radioactive iodine-refractory differentiated thyroid cancer in the elderly. Curr Oncol Rep. 2018;20(10):82.
16. Jegerlehner S, Bulliard JL, Aujesky D, et al. Overdiagnosis and overtreatment of thyroid cancer: a population-based temporal trend study. PLoS One. 2017;12(6):e0179387.
17. Grubey JS, Raji Y, Duke WS, Terris DJ. Outpatient thyroidectomy is safe in the elderly and super-elderly. Laryngoscope. 2018;128(1):290–4.
18. Finnerty BM, Gray KD, Ullmann TM, et al. Frailty is more predictive than age for complications after thyroidectomy for multinodular goiter. World J Surg. 2020;44(6):1876–84.
19. Huang W, Chen YJ, Chen WH. Surgical outcomes of thyroidectomy in geriatric patients aged 80 years and older: a single-center retrospective cohort study. Medicina (Kaunas). 2024;60(9):1383.
20. Goodwin AM, Kurapaty SS, Inglis JE, et al. A meta-analysis of the American college of surgeons risk calculator's predictive accuracy among different surgical sub-specialties. Surg Pract Sci. 2024;16:100238.
21. Kim S, Brooks A, Groban L. Preoperative assessment of the older surgical pa tient: honing in on geriatric syndromes. Clin Interv Aging. 2014;10:13–27.
22. Bible KC, Kebebew E, Brierley J, et al. 2021 American Thyroid Association guidelines for management of patients with anaplastic thyroid cancer. Thyroid. 2021;31(3):337–86.
23. Menon G, Kashyap S, Naing PT, et al. Anaplastic thyroid cancer. 2024 Oct 29. In: StatPearls [Internet]. Treasure Island (FL): StatPearls Publishing; 2025 Jan–.
24. Randle RW, Balentine CJ, Leverson GE, et al. Trends in the presentation, treatment, and survival of patients with medullary thyroid cancer over the past 30 years. Surgery. 2017;161(1):137–46.
25. Sahli ZT, Canner JK, Zeiger MA, Mathur A. Association between age and disease specific mortality in medullary thyroid cancer. Am J Surg. 2021;221(2):478–84.
26. Garberoglio R, Aliberti C, Appetecchia M, et al. Radiofrequency ablation for thyroid nodules: which indications? The first Italian opinion statement. J Ultrasound. 2015;18(4):423–30.
27. Yan L, Li XY, Li Y, Luo Y. Ultrasound-guided radiofrequency ablation versus thyroidectomy for the treatment of benign thyroid nodules in elderly patients: a propensity-matched cohort study. AJNR Am J Neuroradiol. 2023;44(6):693–9.
28. Qian Y, Li Z, Fan C, Huang Y. Comparison of ultrasound-guided microwave ablation, laser ablation, and radiofrequency ablation for the treatment of elderly patients with benign thyroid nodules: a meta-analysis. Exp Gerontol. 2024;191:112425.
29. Hangge PT, Norain A, Butterfield RJ 3rd, et al. Parathyroidectomy in the elderly is beneficial and safe with similar improvements in postoperative bone mineral density. Am J Surg. 2022;224(1 Pt A):147–52.

30. Walker MD, Silverberg SJ. Primary hyperparathyroidism. Nat Rev Endocrinol. 2018;14(2):115–25.
31. Behanova M, Haschka J, Reichardt B, et al. Pelvic fractures - an underestimated problem? Incidence and mortality risk after pelvic fracture in Austria, 2010-2018. J Clin Med. 2022;11(10):2834.
32. Khokar AM, Kuchta KM, Moo-Young TA, et al. Parathyroidectomy is safe in elderly patients: a national surgical quality improvement program study. World J Surg. 2020;44(2):526–36.
33. Habib AR, Katz MH. Parathyroidectomy in elderly individuals with primary hyperparathyroidism: to operate or not to operate. JAMA Intern Med. 2022;182(1):7–8.

Chronic Inflammatory Bowel Disease Surgery

9

Guido Sciaudone, Lucio Selvaggi, and Silvestro Canonico

9.1 Introduction

Inflammatory bowel diseases (IBD), encompassing Crohn's disease (CD) and ulcerative colitis (UC), are lifelong disorders that may arise at any stage of life and are characterized by alternating phases of remission and symptomatic relapse [1–3]. An increasing number of diagnoses are being made in older individuals and, with the progressive aging of the global population, the proportion of elderly IBD patients is expected to rise. Epidemiological projections indicate that by 2030 [4, 5], nearly one-fifth of the United States population will be over 65 years of age, and that 10–15% of IBD patients are diagnosed after the age of 60. Within this subgroup, 25% are aged 70 years or older and approximately 10% are over 80 [6], with a balanced distribution between CD and UC [7, 8] and incidence rates reported up to ~19 per 100,000 individuals [4, 9, 10]. These estimates suggest that, within the next decade, more than one-third of IBD patients will be elderly [11], a trend largely explained by the relatively low disease-related mortality [12]. This chapter focuses on the surgical management of elderly patients with IBD.

G. Sciaudone (✉)
Department of Medicine and Health Sciences V. Tiberio, University of Molise, Campobasso, Italy
e-mail: guido.sciaudone@unimol.it

L. Selvaggi · S. Canonico
Department of Advanced Medical and Surgical Sciences, University of Campania Luigi Vanvitelli, Naples, Italy
e-mail: lucio.selvaggi@unicampania.it; silvestro.canonico@unicampania.it

P. Carcoforo, F. Catena (eds.), *Geriatric Surgery*, Updates in Surgery,
https://doi.org/10.1007/978-3-032-24281-5_9

9.2 Elderly Patients with IBD and Frailty

The definition of "elderly" remains debated in the literature. Chronological age, although commonly adopted, may be misleading as it is influenced by cultural, gender-related, and geographical factors [13]. The World Health Organization identifies elderly individuals as those ≥65 years of age, while geriatric medicine often considers 75–80 years a more appropriate threshold, reflecting the increased prevalence of frailty and age-related comorbidities beyond this age. In Europe, the proportion of people aged ≥80 years has more than tripled over the past five decades, now exceeding 10% of the population [14–16]. The European Crohn's and Colitis Organization (ECCO) [17] defines late-onset IBD as disease onset at ≥60 years, emphasizing that age alone should not guide surgical risk assessment and that surgery should not be delayed when clearly indicated [18, 19]. In these patients, more than others, the assessment of biological reserve and functional status should be considered, as it may be a more accurate predictor of overall health risks. However, frailty in IBD patients remains underexplored in the literature [20, 21].

9.3 Differential Diagnosis

Accurate differential diagnosis is essential in older patients, as IBD can be mistaken for more common conditions. These include complicated diverticular disease with perforation, abscesses, or fistula formation [22] that may mimic IBD or coexist with it [23]; ischemic colitis is often confused with CD [24], NSAID-related diarrhea, post-radiation colitis, and infections such as *Clostridium difficile* [25] colitis must also be considered. Consequently, misdiagnosis occurs in nearly 60% of elderly patients compared to only 15% of younger patients [22, 26, 27]. Furthermore, diagnostic delays [28] may be up to six times longer in the elderly [27, 29, 30].

9.4 Factors Influencing Therapeutic Management

The management of elderly patients with IBD is challenging, as it may be influenced by numerous concurrent factors, including age-related comorbidities such as renal insufficiency, cardiovascular diseases and diabetes [31]. Additional concerns include unpredictable consequences of long-term immunosuppression, heightened infection and cancer risk, polypharmacy, the use of biologic agents [32], malnutrition, reduced physical and cognitive performance, loss of independence, and socioeconomic difficulties [17, 18, 33–35]. Complications related to medical and surgical treatment in elderly IBD patients are poorly documented, although disease progression and the need for surgery appear similar to those in younger cohorts. Importantly, postoperative mortality and complication rates are significantly higher in the elderly [14], yet data remain limited as this population is often excluded from randomized clinical trials [36, 37].

9.5 Surgical Treatment

Although the initial treatment for IBD is primarily medical, many patients, including the elderly, will eventually require surgery due to medical therapy failure [38]. Historically, surgical intervention in older patients was discouraged owing to fears of poor outcomes, but contemporary studies have challenged this view. The main concern is emergency surgery, which carries mortality rates approaching 27% within 30 days. Respiratory infections and sepsis represent leading causes of death in this setting [39]. Additionally, elderly patients also experience more postoperative complications, longer hospital stays, and extended operative times [40–42], partly attributable to comorbid conditions [42]. These observations underscore the need for timely elective surgery, particularly in severe UC, where delays increase the risk of severe complications such as perforation or toxic megacolon and mortality. Early elective intervention, before the patient deteriorates, is associated with better clinical outcomes, making close collaboration between gastroenterologists and surgeons essential [43].

Conversely, recent evidence supports restorative proctocolectomy with ileal pouch-anal anastomosis (IPAA) as a safe option for selected elderly patients and the procedure remains the standard of care for UC. Age should not be considered an absolute contraindication for IPAA, as was previously believed [44], as also emphasized by the American Society of Colon and Rectal Surgeons. Mortality rates following IPAA in elderly patients remain low (<3%) [45].

From a functional perspective, however, the outcomes following IPAA can be less favourable in elderly patients, with more frequent episodes of daytime incontinence and night-time leakage [44]. Moreover, elderly patients are at a higher risk of pouchitis and stenosis of the IPAA in long-term follow-up, although the pouch failure rate does not increase [46]. Surgical success depends largely on preserved sphincter function, intact cognition, and the ability to distinguish between feces and gas [47].

Pellino et al. [1] comparing a group of elderly patients over 70 who underwent restorative proctocolectomy with a younger control group (mean [± SD]: 77.5 [±3.1] vs. 29.9 [±10.6]; $p < 0.0001$) found no statistically significant differences in terms of major complications. However, elderly patients more frequently suffered from dehydration due to stoma output (electrolyte loss from stoma output: 14 [51.8%] vs. 19 [23.4%]; $p = 0.008$). In their experience, younger patients experienced significantly more episodes of small bowel obstruction (17 [20.1%] vs. 1 [3.7%]; $p = 0.04$). No significant differences were observed in bowel control or health-related quality of life, although there was a slight decrease in continence at 3-year follow-up in the elderly group, which did not affect overall satisfaction with the surgery. Similarly, Delaney et al. [47] highlighted this aspect, reporting a high satisfaction rate among elderly patients, with 89% of them stating they would undergo the surgery again and 96% recommending it to others. A 2021 meta-analysis by Pedersen et al. [48], including 13 studies and 1434 patients, reported a complication rate of 47.3% and a 30-day mortality rate of 1.3%. Long-term outcomes such as pouchitis, incontinence, and pouch failure did not differ significantly between patients aged 50–64 and those ≥65 years.

However, in patients with pre-existing incontinence or anorectal dysfunction, IPAA is contraindicated [49], and proctocolectomy with definitive ileostomy should be the procedure of choice. In selected cases with impaired sphincter function, ileorectal anastomosis—no longer recommended in younger UC patients—may still be appropriate in the elderly [50].

Regarding Crohn's disease, advanced age has been suggested as an independent risk factor for postoperative complications [51]. After intestinal resection, recurrence is common, but data on recurrence rates in elderly patients are conflicting. Some studies report significantly higher recurrence compared to younger patients, whereas others suggest lower overall rates but with shorter time to relapse [27]. ECCO [17] notes that the need for surgery in patients with late-onset disease appears to be lower compared to younger patients [52]. In cases requiring surgery for complications related to CD, the procedures, such as abscess drainage, ileal resection, or bowel-sparing surgeries, do not differ between elderly and younger patients [50, 53].

Furthermore, studies indicate that elderly patients adapt well to ileostomy, achieving quality of life comparable to, or even exceeding, that of younger patients [54].

9.6 Conclusions

Chronological age alone should not exclude elderly IBD patients from surgical consideration. Individualized assessment of comorbidities, overall health, and sphincter function is essential. Surgery is frequently undertaken after medical therapy has failed. While emergency procedures carry unacceptably high mortality risks and should be avoided, elective surgery can be performed safely with appropriate patient selection and timing. Although elderly patients may face higher postoperative complication rates and longer hospitalizations, these outcomes are not solely explained by comorbidities. Careful surgical planning and timely intervention are therefore crucial. When tailored to the patient's profile, surgery represents a safe and effective therapeutic option for elderly individuals with IBD.

References

1. Pellino G, Sciaudone G, Candilio G, et al. Complications and functional outcomes of restorative proctocolectomy for ulcerative colitis in the elderly. BMC Surg. 2013;13 Suppl 2(Suppl 2):S9.
2. Pellino G, Sciaudone G, Candilio G, et al. Rectosigmoid stump washout as an alternative to permanent mucous fistula in patients undergoing subtotal colectomy for ulcerative colitis in emergency settings. BMC Surg. 2012;12 Suppl 1(Suppl 1):S31.
3. Pellino G, Sciaudone G, Caserta V, et al. Fatigue in inflammatory bowel diseases: relationship with age and disease activity. Int J Surg. 2014;12 Suppl 2:S60–3.
4. Gisbert JP, Chaparro M. Systematic review with meta-analysis: inflammatory bowel disease in the elderly. Aliment Pharmacol Ther. 2014;39(5):459–77.

5. Ha CY, Katz S. Clinical outcomes and management of inflammatory bowel disease in the older patient. Curr Gastroenterol Rep. 2013;15(2):310.
6. Loftus EV Jr, Silverstein MD, Sandborn WJ, et al. Ulcerative colitis in Olmsted County, Minnesota, 1940-1993: incidence, prevalence, and survival. Gut. 2000;46(3):336–43.
7. Loftus CG, Loftus EV Jr, Harmsen WS, et al. Update on the incidence and prevalence of Crohn's disease and ulcerative colitis in Olmsted County, Minnesota, 1940-2000. Inflamm Bowel Dis. 2007;13(3):254–61.
8. Robertson DJ, Grimm IS. Inflammatory bowel disease in the elderly. Gastroenterol Clin N Am. 2001;30(2):409–26.
9. Singh S, Underwood F, Loftus EV, et al. Sa1769–worldwide incidence of older-onset inflammatory bowel diseases in the 21st century: a systematic review of population-based studies. Gastroenterology. 2019;156(6):S394–5.
10. GBD 2017 Inflammatory Bowel Disease Collaborators. The global, regional, and national burden of inflammatory bowel disease in 195 countries and territories, 1990–2017: a systematic analysis for the Global Burden of Disease Study 2017. Lancet Gastroenterol Hepatol. 2020;5(1):17–30.
11. Coward S, Clement F, Benchimol EI, et al. Past and future burden of inflammatory bowel diseases based on ode ling of population-based data. Gastroenterology. 2019;156(5):1345–53.e4.
12. Pardi DS, Loftus EV Jr, Camilleri M. Treatment of inflammatory bowel disease in the elderly: an update. Drugs Aging. 2002;19(5):355–63.
13. World Health Organization. Men, ageing and health: achieving health across the life span [Internet]. World Health Organization; 2001 [cited 2025 Sept 15]. Available from: https://iris.who.int/handle/10665/66941.
14. Vieujean S, Caron B, Jairath V, et al. Is it time to include older adults in inflammatory bowel disease trials? A call for action. Lancet Healthy Longev. 2022;3(5):e356–66.
15. Bollegala N, Jackson TD, Nguyen GC. Increased postoperative mortality and complications among elderly patients with inflammatory bowel diseases: an analysis of the national surgical quality improvement program cohort. Clin Gastroenterol Hepatol. 2016;14(9):1274–81.
16. Nguyen GC, Elnahas A, Jackson TD. The impact of preoperative steroid use on short-term outcomes following surgery for inflammatory bowel disease. J Crohns Colitis. 2014;8(12):1661–7.
17. Sturm A, Maaser C, Mendall M, et al. European Crohn's and Colitis Organisation topical review on IBD in the elderly. J Crohns Colitis. 2017;11(3):263–73.
18. Charpentier C, Salleron J, Savoye G, et al. Natural history of elderly-onset inflammatory bowel disease: a population-based cohort study. Gut. 2014;63(3):423–32.
19. Nimmons D, Limdi JK. Elderly patients and inflammatory bowel disease. World J Gastrointest Pharmacol Ther. 2016;7(1):51–65.
20. Hoogendijk EO, Afilalo J, Ensrud KE, et al. Frailty: implications for clinical practice and public health. Lancet. 2019;394(10206):1365–75.
21. Qian AS, Nguyen NH, Elia J, et al. Frailty is independently associated with mortality and readmission in hospitalized patients with inflammatory bowel diseases. Clin Gastroenterol Hepatol. 2021;19(10):2054–63.e14.
22. Katz S, Pardi DS. Inflammatory bowel disease of the elderly: frequently asked questions (FAQs). Am J Gastroenterol. 2011;106(11):1889–97.
23. Gabrielli F, Di Gioia F, Di Sibio T, et al. [Crohn's disease in the elderly]. Ann Ital Chir. 1995;66(6):851–6.
24. Montoro MA, Brandt LJ, Santolaria S, et al. Clinical patterns and outcomes of ischaemic colitis: results of the working group for the Study of Ischaemic Colitis in Spain (CIE study). Scand J Gastroenterol. 2011;46(2):236–46.
25. Ananthakrishnan AN, McGinley EL, Binion DG. Excess hospitalisation burden associated with Clostridium difficile in patients with inflammatory bowel disease. Gut. 2008;57(2):205–10.
26. Foxworthy DM, Wilson JA. Crohn's disease in the elderly. Prolonged delay in diagnosis. J Am Geriatr Soc. 1985;33(7):492–5.
27. Wagtmans MJ, Verspaget HW, Lamers CB, van Hogezand RA. Crohn's disease in the elderly: a comparison with young adults. J Clin Gastroenterol. 1998;27(2):129–33.

28. Pellino G, Sciaudone G, Selvaggi F, Riegler G. Delayed diagnosis is influenced by the clinical pattern of Crohn's disease and affects treatment outcomes and quality of life in the long term: a cross-sectional study of 361 patients in Southern Italy. Eur J Gastroenterol Hepatol. 2015;27(2):175–81.
29. Harper PC, McAuliffe TL, Beeken WL. Crohn's disease in the elderly. A statistical comparison with younger patients matched for sex and duration of disease. Arch Intern Med. 1986;146(4):753–5.
30. Zimmerman J, Gavish D, Rachmilewitz D. Early and late onset ulcerative colitis: distinct clinical features. J Clin Gastroenterol. 1985;7(6):492–8.
31. Fuschillo G, Celentano V, Rottoli M, et al. Influence of diabetes mellitus on inflammatory bowel disease course and treatment outcomes. A systematic review with meta-analysis. Dig Liver Dis. 2023;55(5):580–6.
32. Selvaggi F, Pellino G, Canonico S, Sciaudone G. Effect of preoperative biologic drugs on complications and function after restorative proctocolectomy with primary ileal pouch formation: systematic review and meta-analysis. Inflamm Bowel Dis. 2015;21(1):79–92.
33. Lakatos PL, David G, Pandur T, et al. IBD in the elderly population: results from a population-based study in western Hungary, 1977-2008. J Crohns Colitis. 2011;5(1):5–13.
34. Ha CY, Katz S. Clinical implications of ageing for the management of IBD. Nat Rev Gastroenterol Hepatol. 2014;11(2):128–38.
35. Juneja M, Baidoo L, Schwartz MB, et al. Geriatric inflammatory bowel disease: phenotypic presentation, treatment patterns, nutritional status, outcomes, and comorbidity. Dig Dis Sci. 2012;57(9):2408–15.
36. Cherubini A, Del Signore S, Ouslander J, et al. Fighting against age discrimination in clinical trials. J Am Geriatr Soc. 2010;58(9):1791–6.
37. Kochar B, Kalasapudi L, Ufere NN, et al. Systematic review of inclusion and analysis of older adults in randomized controlled trials of medications used to treat inflammatory bowel diseases. Inflamm Bowel Dis. 2021;27(9):1541–3.
38. Carr N, Schofield PF. Inflammatory bowel disease in the older patient. Br J Surg. 1982;69(4):223–5.
39. Ikeuchi H, Uchino M, Matsuoka H, et al. Prognosis following emergency surgery for ulcerative colitis in elderly patients. Surg Today. 2014;44(1):39–43.
40. Ananthakrishnan AN, EL MG, Binion DG. Inflammatory bowel disease in the elderly is associated with worse outcomes: a national study of hospitalizations. Inflamm Bowel Dis. 2009;15(2):182–9.
41. Murata Y, Ueoka K, Suzuki T, et al. An experiment of acute fulminant severe ulcerative colitis in a 75- year-old male – a case report and a consideration of the surgical treatment of elderly patients with severe ulcerative colitis. Nihon Geka Gakkai Zasshi. 1987;88(2):216–21.
42. Page MJ, Poritz LS, Kunselman SJ, Koltun WA. Factors affecting surgical risk in elderly patients with inflammatory bowel disease. J Gastrointest Surg. 2002;6(4):606–13.
43. Sousa P, Bertani L, Rodrigues C. Management of inflammatory bowel disease in the elderly: a review. Dig Liver Dis. 2023;55(8):1001–9.
44. del Val JH. Old-age inflammatory bowel disease onset: a different problem? World J Gastroenterol. 2011;17(22):2734–9.
45. Almogy G, Sachar DB, Bodian CA, Greenstein AJ. Surgery for ulcerative colitis in elderly persons: changes in indications for surgery and outcome over time. Arch Surg. 2001;136(12):1396–400.
46. Chapman JR, Larson DW, Wolff BG, et al. Ileal pouch-anal anastomosis: does age at the time of surgery affect outcome? Arch Surg. 2005;140(6):534–9.
47. Delaney CP, Fazio VW, Remzi FH, et al. Prospective, age-related analysis of surgical results, functional outcome, and quality of life after ileal pouch-anal anastomosis. Ann Surg. 2003;238(2):221–8.
48. Pedersen KE, Jia X, Holubar SD, et al. Ileal pouch-anal anastomosis in the elderly: a systematic review and meta-analysis. Color Dis. 2021;23(8):2062–74.

49. Farouk R, Pemberton JH, Wolff BG, et al. Functional outcomes after ileal pouch-anal anastomosis for chronic ulcerative colitis. Ann Surg. 2000;231(6):919–26.
50. Stallmach A, Hagel S, Gharbi A, et al. Medical and surgical therapy of inflammatory bowel disease in the elderly – prospects and complications. J Crohns Colitis. 2011;5(3):177–88.
51. Molodecky NA, Soon IS, Rabi DM, et al. Increasing incidence and prevalence of the inflammatory bowel diseases with time, based on systematic review. Gastroenterology. 2012;142(1):46–54.e42.
52. Tremaine WJ, Timmons LJ, Loftus EV Jr, et al. Age at onset of inflammatory bowel disease and the risk of surgery for non-neoplastic bowel disease. Aliment Pharmacol Ther. 2007;25(12):1435–41.
53. Polito JM 2nd, Childs B, Mellits ED, et al. Crohn's disease: influence of age at diagnosis on site and clinical type of disease. Gastroenterology. 1996;111(3):580–6.
54. Stryker SJ, Pemberton JH, Zinsmeister AR. Long-term results of ileostomy in older patients. Dis Colon Rectum. 1985;28(11):844–6.

Pancreatic Surgery

10

Giovanna Di Meo, Piercarmine Panzera, and Mario Testini

10.1 Introduction

Pancreatic malignancy (PM) remains one of the leading causes of cancer-related mortality in Western countries. Pancreatic cancer (PC) incidence increases with age, with approximately 70% of patients being 65 years or older at the time of diagnosis. The mean age at diagnosis is 72 years; about 29% of cases occur in patients aged 75–84 years, and 13% in those aged ≥85 years. The proportion of elderly patients (EPs) in Western countries is steadily rising, representing the fastest-growing segment of the population. This demographic shift is progressively increasing the number of EPs presenting with pancreatic or periampullary malignancy and, consequently, the number of complex surgical candidates in this age group.

This population is particularly vulnerable to malnutrition, often related to reduced dietary intake and age-related physiological changes of the gastrointestinal tract. Similar functional declines are well described in secretory organs such as the liver, kidney, and intestine. The pancreas itself, a metabolically active organ essential for nutrient processing, undergoes progressive morphological and functional alterations with age. Pancreatic volume increases until adulthood, stabilizes between 20 and 60 years, and subsequently declines due to parenchymal loss, fibrosis, reduced perfusion, and atrophy. These changes may impair exocrine function even in otherwise healthy EPs. Indeed, pancreatic exocrine insufficiency, defined by fecal elastase-1 levels <200 μg/g stool, is observed in approximately 5% of people older than 70 years and in 10% of those over 80 years. Pancreatic exocrine insufficiency can lead itself to maldigestion, malnutrition, and deficiencies in fat-soluble vitamins, with downstream consequences such as reduced bone mineral density due to impaired vitamin D absorption. Clinical manifestations may include steatorrhea,

G. Di Meo (✉) · P. Panzera · M. Testini
Department of Precision and Regenerative Medicine and Ionian Area (DiMePre-J), University of Bari Aldo Moro, Bari, Italy
e-mail: giovanna.dimeo@policlinico.ba.it; mario.testini@uniba.it

P. Carcoforo, F. Catena (eds.), *Geriatric Surgery*, Updates in Surgery,
https://doi.org/10.1007/978-3-032-24281-5_10

diarrhea, abdominal discomfort, and weight loss, although symptoms are often subtle. As a consequence, the onset of PM in an already metabolically compromised organ, compounds the burden of malnutrition and contributing to the progressive deterioration of the patient's clinical condition.

In this context, surgical decision-making in EPs with pancreatic or periampullary malignancy is particularly challenging. Pancreatic resection entails considerable physiological stress, and the risk-benefit assessment is more complex compared to younger patients. Frailty, comorbidities (e.g., cardiovascular, respiratory, and metabolic disorders), and reduced physiological reserves increase vulnerability to perioperative morbidity and mortality. Age-related declines in hepatic and renal function further compromise drug metabolism and excretion, raising the risk of adverse effects and postoperative complications. Historically, these factors contributed to the perception that pancreatic resection in EPs, especially octogenarians, was associated with prohibitive risks.

However, advances in perioperative care, anesthesia, oncological treatments, and the centralization of pancreatic surgery (PS) in high-volume centers have substantially improved postoperative outcomes. Several studies now report that EPs, including those ≥70 years, are increasingly undergoing pancreaticoduodenectomy (PD) with acceptable outcomes. Moreover, pancreatic resection has been associated with improved overall survival (OS) compared to non-operative management in selected EPs with resectable disease.

Nevertheless, outcomes in octogenarians remain debated. Although PS has been shown to be safe and feasible in experienced centers, reported morbidity and mortality rates are higher than in younger cohorts—approximately 34.9% and 13.2%, respectively, with a longer average hospital stay. Furthermore, less than 50% of EPs receive adjuvant chemotherapy postoperatively, potentially limiting survival benefits. Median OS following pancreatic resection in patients aged ≥80 years has been reported at 17.6 months, comparable to younger populations. Data on postoperative quality of life (QOL) in this group are limited, but available reports emphasize the frequent need for rehabilitation and health support services, underscoring the frailty of this population.

In summary, the combination of population aging, advances in surgical and perioperative care, and evidence of improved outcomes in EPs has prompted growing interest in the safety and feasibility of PS in this demographic. While surgery in octogenarians can be performed safely in high-volume centers, it remains associated with increased morbidity, mortality, and healthcare needs. Careful patient selection and comprehensive geriatric assessment are essential to balance surgical risks with potential long-term benefits, particularly in terms of survival and QOL [1].

10.2 Surgery

10.2.1 Indications

The optimal treatment for PM is surgical resection combined with systemic chemotherapy. Despite advances in perioperative management, PS remains one of the most complex procedures in abdominal surgery, carrying substantial risks of morbidity and mortality. PD is particularly demanding and associated with specific complications, including postoperative pancreatic fistula (POPF), post-pancreatectomy hemorrhage (PPH), and delayed gastric emptying (DGE). Other procedures, such as distal pancreatectomy (DP) and total pancreatectomy (TP) also require extensive resections, though they are generally associated with lower complication rates compared with PD [2, 3].

In clinical practice, malignant disease accounts for the vast majority of pancreatic resections (89.8%). Among these, pancreatic ductal adenocarcinoma (PDAC) represents the most frequent tumor (74.6%), followed by periampullary carcinoma (11.6%) and cholangiocarcinoma (6.6%). Other malignant indications include neuroendocrine tumors, degenerate intraductal papillary mucinous neoplasms (IPMNs) and, less commonly, secondary pancreatic tumors. In contrast, benign or borderline lesions constitute only 10.2% of resections, most often involving IPMNs (39.1%), cystic neoplasms (20.3%), and neuroendocrine tumors (9.4%).

The management of IPMNs poses unique challenges, particularly in EPs. QOL studies in non-IPMN post-pancreatectomy patients suggest that most functional domains recover to preoperative levels within 3 months; however, the presence of malignancy is associated with poorer long-term outcomes, with diminished QOL reported at 2 years. While resection remains the standard of care for IPMNs meeting surgical criteria, non-operative management may be appropriate in selected patients, especially those with significant comorbidities or limited life expectancy, in whom overall and disease-specific survival appears comparable between surgery and observation. Conversely, patients without prohibitive comorbidities should be offered resection, with thorough counseling regarding the risks of malignancy, the potential for surgical complications, and the expected survival outcomes for both invasive and non-invasive disease.

10.2.2 Selection of Surgical Candidates

The selection of surgical candidates and the decision between neoadjuvant therapy and upfront surgery are crucial in the management of PC, requiring consideration of both patient-related and disease-related factors.

Several studies highlight the prognostic role of comorbidities in EPs. A U.S. national analysis showed worse survival in those over 80 years, particularly with ≥2 comorbidities, while a National Cancer Center study found surgery improved survival but confirmed the comorbidity index as an independent predictor [4, 5].

Similarly, survival benefits in octogenarians have been demonstrated only when patients were mentally and physically fit with favorable operative risk scores. These findings support the use of a Comprehensive Geriatric Assessment (CGA) to identify impairments not captured by routine evaluation and to better predict short- and long-term outcomes. Consensus guidelines recommend CGA domains such as functional, nutritional, and psychological status, social support, comorbidity, polypharmacy, and cognition, which are also relevant for predicting chemotherapy tolerance [6].

Disease factors further influence outcomes. EPs with resectable disease may achieve prognoses comparable to younger cohorts, but survival is poorer in borderline or locally advanced cancers, largely due to lower completion rates of adjuvant chemotherapy. Neoadjuvant therapy may mitigate this limitation: the RESPECT study and others have shown comparable resectability and survival between EPs and younger patients after neoadjuvant therapy, and recent data suggest that this is both safe and effective in selected EPs, supporting calls for randomized trials [7–9].

Finally, decision-making must account for the risks of surgery, potential loss of function, and diminished QOL, while respecting individual values and preferences. Given the lack of high-quality evidence and the underrepresentation of older adults in clinical trials, traditional informed consent is insufficient. A shared decision-making model is recommended to integrate patient priorities with clinical judgment, aiming to reduce unwanted interventions, postoperative distress, and to ensure value-concordant care.

10.2.3 Surgical Approach

The introduction of minimally invasive pancreatic surgery (MIPR), including laparoscopic and robotic techniques, has expanded opportunities to reduce surgical trauma in EPs. These approaches are associated with reduced intraoperative blood loss, shorter hospital stays, and potentially faster recovery, while maintaining oncological radicality.

Evidence from the Italian Association for Pancreatology (AISP) multicenter study, which analyzed 780 EPs across 25 centers, demonstrated the feasibility and safety of MIPR. Compared with open pancreatic resection (OPR), MIPR was associated with lower overall morbidity (30.7% vs. 42.3%), fewer severe complications (15.3% vs. 23.9%), and shorter hospitalization (median 11 vs. 13 days), without compromising oncologic outcomes such as R0 resection rates, lymph node yield, or survival (33.5 vs. 29.6 months). However, patient selection bias was evident, as MIPR patients were generally younger, fitter, and had smaller tumors. After adjustment, survival and oncologic outcomes were equivalent between MIPR and OPR.

A meta-analysis by Ballarin et al. including 1378 patients confirmed that MIPR is feasible in selected EPs. While these patients had higher intraoperative blood loss and perioperative mortality, their conversion rates, overall complications, POPF, DGE, and oncologic parameters were comparable to younger patients. Similarly, a large retrospective study by Shyr et al. showed that robotic resection is technically feasible in octogenarians, although mortality, DGE, and biliary leaks were more frequent in this subgroup. These findings emphasize the importance of rigorous patient selection and careful perioperative assessment [10].

The learning curve remains a key limitation, particularly for laparoscopic or robotic PD, which requires substantial experience. In EPs, this challenge is compounded by reduced physiological reserve, anatomical changes, and increased vulnerability to complications. Consequently, MIPR in this population should be performed only in high-volume centers by highly experienced surgeons, supported by structured training, mentorship, and simulation-based programs that incorporate geriatric considerations.

From a health-economics perspective, MIPR entails higher upfront costs due to longer operative times and specialized technology, but these may be offset by shorter hospital stays, lower complication rates, and faster recovery—factors particularly relevant for EPs with limited physiological reserve and higher dependency risks. When performed in high-volume centers, emerging data suggest MIPR can be cost-effective in older adults through reduced postoperative resource utilization and lower readmission rates [11, 12].

10.2.4 Perioperative Care

Once the decision to proceed with surgery has been made, perioperative management tailored to the elderly population becomes essential. Prehabilitation, particularly relevant for older cancer patients, aims to optimize physiological reserve before surgery, thereby reducing recovery time and postoperative complications. Core elements of prehabilitation include cardiovascular and skeletal muscle training, nutritional optimization, psychological support, and medical management of comorbidities. While its benefits have been demonstrated in several major surgical settings, evidence in PS remains limited. Nonetheless, given the frequent presence of cachexia, sarcopenia, and nutritional impairment in PM, EPs may particularly benefit from structured prehabilitation programs designed to improve nutritional status and cardiorespiratory fitness.

Postoperatively, geriatric-specific care should follow a multidisciplinary approach. The applicability of enhanced recovery after surgery (ERAS®) pathways in EPs undergoing pancreatic resction remains an area of active investigation. Updated ERAS® guidelines and meta-analyses report favorable effects, including reduced hospital stay after PD in older patients, although further randomized controlled trials are needed to confirm their efficacy. Importantly, increasing age has not been associated with poorer ERAS® compliance or worse outcomes, suggesting that ERAS® protocols are both safe and feasible in this population.

Overall, both prehabilitation and ERAS® appear promising for optimizing surgical outcomes in EPs with PM. Tailored, multimodal programs that account for geriatric-specific vulnerabilities are needed to maximize benefit. While standard surgical principles apply to carefully selected EPs, extensive resections that substantially increase operative risk should be avoided, particularly in very EPs with locally advanced disease. Personalized perioperative care thus represents a key strategy to improve outcomes in this high-risk population.

10.3 Early Outcomes

10.3.1 Mortality and Morbidity

Population-based cohort studies have demonstrated that in-hospital mortality following pancreatic resection increases with age, particularly among patients aged 80 years or older. Data from the American College of Surgery- National Surgical Quality Improvement Program (ACS-NSQIP) database, analyzing 17,835 patients undergoing PD, demonstrated higher 30-day mortality (5.9% vs. 2.8%) and severe complications (35.8% vs. 28.7%) in patients ≥80 years compared to those <80. The most common complications following pancreatic resection include POPF, DGE and cardiopulmonary complications. Also the rate of reoperation is higher among elder patients.

However, these findings are largely driven by the higher prevalence of comorbidities in the older group. Notably, major surgery-related complications—such as POPF, DGE, and PPH—do not significantly differ between EPs and younger patients. Conversely, respiratory complications are more prevalent in the EPs, corroborating existing literature that medical complications are more frequent in this population compared to younger individuals. This is supported by multicenter retrospective analyses which utilized propensity score matching to balance patient characteristics. Their results indicated no significant differences between EPs (≥80 years) and younger patients in mortality, major surgical complications, POPF grades B and C, medical complications, reoperation rates, or length of hospital stay, provided that patients were appropriately selected. Moreover, an American Society of Anesthesiologists (ASA) score ≥3 emerged as an independent predictor of major complications, emphasizing the critical role of thorough preoperative assessment.

The extent of surgery is a critical determinant of outcomes. Patients requiring portal vein resection have significantly worse outcomes, emphasizing the importance of tailoring surgical indication and avoiding extensive resections in this age group.

In conclusion, although pancreatic resection in EPs is associated with increased risks, these outcomes are largely influenced by the presence of comorbidities and patient frailty. With careful patient selection, comprehensive multidisciplinary management, and experienced surgical teams, comparable postoperative outcomes to those of younger patients can be achieved, thereby providing EPs with a viable therapeutic option [13].

10.3.2 Functional Recovery

Beyond mortality and morbidity, functional recovery represent crucial endpoints for EPs undergoing PS. This population is particularly vulnerable to delayed convalescence, prolonged dependency, and reduced postoperative resilience. Studies have shown that older adults are more likely to require discharge to rehabilitation facilities or skilled nursing care rather than directly home, underscoring the long-term impact of surgery beyond the immediate postoperative phase. Preoperative sarcopenia has emerged as a key prognostic factor. Identified in over 40% of EPs, sarcopenia is strongly associated with impaired functional recovery, increased length of HS, and higher rates of postoperative complications. Structured rehabilitation protocols and early mobilization have been shown to mitigate some of these adverse effects, facilitating earlier return to independence and reducing hospital readmission rates.

10.4 Late Outcomes

Reported survival after pancreatic resection in EPs varies considerably across studies, reflecting differences in patient selection, surgical techniques, and adjuvant chemotherapy use, with one-year survival rates ranging from 50% to 75.7%, and five-year survival rates ranging from 0% to 46%. These wide variations underscore the heterogeneity of surgical indications and perioperative care among elderly populations. Overall, surgery is not consistently identified as a positive prognostic factor for very EPs, yet it remains the only chance for achieving survival beyond 3 years in this age group. Surgical extent influences long-term outcomes. While surgery can provide meaningful survival, aggressive procedures such as PD combined with portal vein resection should be considered with caution in the very elderly. OS in EPs is consistently shorter than in younger cohorts. This discrepancy has been attributed in part to lower utilization of adjuvant chemotherapy in the elderly, despite clear evidence that it improves survival.

Beyond survival, QOL is a critical consideration in EPs undergoing major surgery. Unfortunately, QOL outcomes have been underreported in the literature. Fatigue is the most common symptom in the first 6 months after surgery; however, QOL scores improved rapidly thereafter, returning to near-normal levels within months. It has been reported that patients aged 80 years or older are more frequently discharged to nursing facilities compared to younger patients, mainly due to the need for rehabilitation programs addressing both physical activity and digestive function [14, 15].

10.5 Adjuvant Chemotherapy

Adjuvant chemotherapy has been shown to improve survival following curative-intent pancreatic resection, but EPs are less likely to receive or complete treatment. Several single-center studies illustrate this trend. When chemotherapy is omitted, both OS and disease-free survival (DFS) seem significantly reduced compared to younger patients. Thus, where feasible, efforts should be made to provide adjuvant chemotherapy, ideally supported by geriatric assessment to guide patient selection. Treatment-related toxicity is a major concern in the elderly. Age-related pharmacokinetic and pharmacodynamic changes, reduced organ function, and polypharmacy increase the risk of adverse events. Hematologic toxicity (neutropenia, anemia, thrombocytopenia) and gastrointestinal toxicity (diarrhea, mucositis, nausea) are particularly common. In pooled analyses, EPs receiving combination chemotherapy experienced higher rates of grade ≥3 toxicity compared with younger cohorts, often leading to dose reductions, treatment delays, or early discontinuation. Nevertheless, studies suggest that fit EPs with preserved performance status and limited comorbidities can tolerate combination regimens, albeit often requiring modified doses. The use of CGA tools, such as the G-8 or Charlson Comorbidity Index, has been shown to better predict tolerability than chronological age alone. In the postoperative setting, single-agent gemcitabine or 5-fluorouracil plus leucovorin is often preferred. Modified regimens (e.g., reduced-dose mFOLFIRINOX [folinic acid, fluorouracil, irinotecan, oxaliplatin]) may be offered to carefully selected octogenarians with excellent performance status, but caution is warranted.

10.6 System Approach

EPs undergoing PD face increased morbidity and mortality due to reduced physiological reserve ("homeostenosis"), which impairs recovery and heightens the risk of failure to rescue. Frailty, rather than chronological age alone, has emerged as a more accurate predictor of postoperative outcomes.

Textbook Outcome (TO) provides a composite measure of surgical quality, defined for PD as the absence of major complications (POPF, PPH, bile leak, Clavien-Dindo ≥III), in-hospital/30-day mortality, and 30-day readmission. While widely applied in hepatopancreatobiliary surgery, its relevance in the elderly remains underexplored. A recent dual-center analysis of 222 patients ≥70 years showed that 54.5% achieved TO, though rates declined with age (57.1% at 70–74 vs. 35.0% in octogenarians). Independent predictors of TO failure included age ≥80, ASA ≥2, and non-PDAC or non-distal cholangiocarcinoma pathology, underscoring the impact of comorbidity burden and advanced age [16].

Structured geriatric care models, such as Duke's Perioperative Optimization of Senior Health program, have demonstrated reductions in complications, readmissions, and length of hospital stay, highlighting the value of tailored perioperative strategies. Yet EPs remain underrepresented in clinical research, comprising only ~7% of randomized trials, limiting evidence-based guidance.

Among the guidelines, the Japan Pancreas Society uniquely addresses patients ≥80 years, recommending surgery when both clinical condition and patient preference allow. Similarly, a 2019 consensus from geriatric oncology and hepatopancreatobiliary experts emphasized multimodal, individualized strategies integrating medical risk, autonomy, and shared decision-making.

10.7 Conclusion

Although EPs are at higher risk of morbidity, mortality, and reduced long-term survival, surgical safety has improved substantially over time. Careful patient selection, patient-centered decision-making, prehabilitation, and structured postoperative geriatric care—including ERAS® protocols—can enhance outcomes. Surgeons must adopt a geriatric-focused approach, supported by institutional systems and academic initiatives, to ensure that EPs, when appropriately selected and optimized, can undergo PS with principles comparable to those applied in younger cohorts.

References

1. Di Meo G, Prete FP, Fischetti E, et al. Benchmarking in pancreatic surgery: a systematic review of metric development and validation. Updat Surg. 2024;76(6):2103–28.
2. Kim SW. Surgical management for elderly patients with pancreatic cancer. Ann Surg Treat Res. 2023;105(2):63–8.
3. Ingaldi C, Minghetti M, D'ambra V, et al. Pancreatic cancer resection in the elderly: state of the art, and future challenges. A systematic review. Minerva Surg. 2025;80(2):138–49.
4. Riall TS, Reddy DM, Nealon WH, Goodwin JS. The effect of age on short-term outcomes after pancreatic resection: a population-based study. Ann Surg. 2008;248(3):459–67.
5. Satoi S, Yamamoto T, Uchida K, et al. Optimal treatment for octogenarians with resectable and borderline resectable pancreatic ductal adenocarcinoma: a multicenter retrospective study. Pancreas. 2020;49(6):837–44.
6. Hartog M, Beishuizen SJE, Togo R, et al. Comprehensive geriatric assessment, treatment decisions, and outcomes in older patients eligible for pancreatic surgery. J Surg Oncol. 2024;130(8):1643–53.
7. Weniger M, Moir J, Damm M, et al. Neoadjuvant therapy in elderly patients receiving FOLFIRINOX or gemcitabine/nab-paclitaxel for borderline resectable or locally advanced pancreatic cancer is feasible and lead to a similar oncological outcome compared to non-aged patients - results of the RESPECT-study. Surg Oncol. 2020;35:285–97.
8. Rieser CJ, Zenati M, Narayanan S, et al. Optimal management of resectable pancreatic head cancer in the elderly patient: does neoadjuvant therapy offer a survival benefit? Ann Surg Oncol. 2021;28(11):6264–72.
9. Cooper AB, Holmes HM, des Bordes JK, et al. Role of neoadjuvant therapy in the multimodality treatment of older patients with pancreatic cancer. J Am Coll Surg. 2014;219(1):111–20.
10. Ballarin R, Esposito G, Guerrini GP, et al. Minimally invasive pancreaticoduodenectomy in elderly versus younger patients: a meta-analysis. Cancers (Basel). 2024;16(2):323.
11. Bartos A, Mărgărit S, Bocse H, et al. Laparoscopic pancreatoduodenectomy in elderly patients: a systematic review and meta-analysis. Life (Basel). 2022;12(11):1810.
12. Park HM, Park SJ, Han SS, Kim SH. Surgery for elderly patients with resectable pancreatic cancer, a comparison with nonsurgical treatments: a retrospective study outcomes of resectable pancreatic cancer. BMC Cancer. 2019;19(1):1090.
13. Quero G, Pecorelli N, Paiella S, et al. Pancreaticoduodenectomy in octogenarians: the importance of "biological age" on clinical outcomes. Surg Oncol. 2022;40:101688.
14. Finlayson E, Fan Z, Birkmeyer JD. Outcomes in octogenarians undergoing high-risk cancer operation: a national study. J Am Coll Surg. 2007;205(6):729–34.
15. Sho M, Murakami Y, Kawai M, et al. Prognosis after surgical treatment for pancreatic cancer in patients aged 80 years or older: a multicenter study. J Hepatobiliary Pancreat Sci. 2016;23(3):188–97.
16. Mocchegiani F, Benedetti Cacciaguerra A, Wakabayashi T, et al. Textbook outcome following pancreaticoduodenectomy in elderly patients: age-stratified analysis and predictive factors. Updat Surg. 2025;77(5):1501–11.

Surgical Management of Full-Thickness Rectal Prolapse in the Elderly Patient

11

Francesco Gabrielli, Angelo Guttadauro, Matteo Maternini, Nicoletta Pecora, and Dorotea Confalonieri

11.1 Epidemiology and Etiology

Though uncommon, full-thickness rectal prolapse (FTRP) is a debilitating condition that diminishes the quality of life. Its incidence in the general population is 0.2–0.4% and 1% in those aged over 65 years [1, 2], and it increases with advancing age: 21.7% in the seventh decade, 31.7% in the eight decade, and 20% in the ninth decade, as observed by M.R. Keighley in 120 cases [3]. It is more prevalent among older women than older men [1].

Risk factors for the development of FTRP include multi-parity by vaginal birth and a history of pelvic surgery, neurological or psychiatric disorders (stroke, spina bifida, dementia), and cystic fibrosis. Contributing factors are bowel dysfunction (irritable bowel syndrome, chronic constipation, diarrhea) or bowel habits such as chronic excessive straining during defecation. In 30% of cases, it may be associated with rectal functional disorders (puborectal muscle syndrome, sphincter dyssynergia, descending perineum syndrome) or other perineal anomalies (genital or pelvic organ prolapse, enterocele, sigmoidocele).

The fact that over one-hundred different procedures for rectal prolapse repair have been described to date reveals how little we actually know about the etiology [4–6]. Factors predisposing to the development of rectal prolapse include sigmoid colon redundancy, abnormally deep pouch of Douglas, weakening and collapse of the anatomical structures derived from the pelvic fascia (lateral rectal ligaments),

F. Gabrielli (✉) · A. Guttadauro · M. Maternini
Department of General Surgery, University of Milan Bicocca, Zucchi Hospital, Monza, Italy
e-mail: francesco.gabrielli52@gmail.com; angelo.guttadauro@unimib.it

N. Pecora
Department of General Surgery, University of Milan Bicocca, Milan, Italy
e-mail: nicoletta.pecora@unimib.it

D. Confalonieri
Department of General Surgery, University of Insubria, Zucchi Hospital, Monza, Italy

P. Carcoforo, F. Catena (eds.), *Geriatric Surgery*, Updates in Surgery,
https://doi.org/10.1007/978-3-032-24281-5_11

more obtuse anorectal angle at rest, and congenital or progressive weakening of the muscles of the pelvic diaphragm (levator ani muscle) [3]). A main causal role in its development has been attributed to intussusception [5]. A unifying explanation proposed for its pathogenesis is that the prolapse begins cranially as an internal or occult sigmoidorectal or high rectorectal prolapse that then invaginates distally to form a rectoanal prolapse that eventually protrudes externally, becoming a FTRP, conventionally defined as rectal prolapse if the segment is up to 5–6 cm in length or sigmoidorectal if longer. As it continues to descend, an internal rectal prolapse can deform the anterior peritoneal wall, giving rise to rectocele: intussusception and rectocele thus contribute to dyschezia caused by obstructed defecation [6].

In 15–65% of cases, FTRP is associated with constipation; in 75% of patients, stretching of the nerve fibers and the anal sphincters leads to a variable degree of incontinence [3, 4, 7], which is more prevalent in patients over 60 years of age and especially in the multiparous (85% of cases) [3].

11.2 Surgical Therapy

Symptom severity and the risk of complications are indications for surgical treatment in elderly patients, too. Medical management is reserved for very frail patients, in whom palliative treatment of functional symptoms is focused on correct diet, Kegel exercises to strengthen the pelvic floor muscles, or biofeedback therapy to improve sphincter control [8].

11.3 Abdominal Procedures

11.3.1 Traditional Rectopexy

For nearly 30 years, traditional rectopexy procedures were the most widely used techniques and yielded good outcomes for prolapse repair [9–11]. In the Wells procedure (posterior sling rectopexy), a mesh is anchored to the sacrum and wrapped 270° posterolaterally around the rectum [12], while in the Orr-Loygue procedure two prosthetic polytetrafluoroethylene (PTFE) strips are fixed to the anterolateral surface of the rectum and back to the sacral promontory [13]. The Ripstein procedure involved a mesh encircling the rectum entirely [14] but was subsequently abandoned because of the risk of occlusion from stenotic scarring. Simple rectopexy using non-absorbable sutures instead of a mesh for fixation to the presacral fascia from 1–2 to 4–5 cm below the sacral promontory has been shown to be non-inferior to rectopexy with mesh [15]. Most commonly performed under general anesthesia, rectopexy can also be carried out under peridural anesthesia in selected patients.

In both male and female patients, the rectum is mobilized to the tip of the coccyx posteriorly and anteriorly to expose the plane of the levator muscles. Debate continues about whether or not to resect the lateral rectal ligaments, with some surgeons arguing that the ligaments are weakened in rectal prolapse [3] and the majority maintaining that ligament resection leads to parasympathetic denervation, resulting in the onset or worsening of constipation. On the other hand, while sparing the ligaments may reduce the risk of constipation, it increases the risk of prolapse recurrence [16, 17]. Furthermore, ligament resection may also affect colon transit time and increase the frequency of bowel movement, reducing rectal elasticity and capacity [18].

Rectopexy has been considered the gold standard of surgical treatment for rectal prolapse since it is associated with a recurrence rate of less than 5% (mean rate, 2–3%) [3, 4, 7, 9, 19–22]. The operative mortality rate ranges between 0% and 7% but remains acceptable on average. Morbidity ranges more widely (0–20%) [3, 7, 9, 10, 19–22]: the major complications are bleeding (even life-threatening in cases of sacral vein lesion), prosthesis infection producing pelvic abscess, stenotic scarring, and erosion fistulas. While prosthesis-related complications (infection, stenosis, erosion) are obviously absent in simple rectopexy, other complications are similar to those seen after rectopexy with use of a mesh [3, 9, 10].

Incontinence after surgery is improved in about 60% of patients [3]. Since improvement may not be noted until at least 6 months after the operation, particularly in elderly patients, other therapeutic options for treating incontinence, especially further surgery, should be delayed accordingly. Studies seeking to identify predicting factors of functional improvement based on preoperative examinations have found that patients presenting with low basal pressure and maximum squeeze pressure have a higher probability of remaining incontinent after rectopexy [3]. Morphologic evaluation with CT and MR imaging of the perineal musculature has shown that impairment of sphincter and levator ani muscle function can be useful for diagnosis and prognosis [23].

Improvement in constipation after rectopexy ranges widely across studies, with some reporting improvement in 15–80% of patients and others noting new onset or worsening of constipation in 15–50% [4, 7, 9, 10, 22, 24–27]. Patients with pre-existing constipation have a greater probability of not experiencing improvement or even worsening of the condition after surgery [3]. Other reasons for failed improvement are pre-existing colonic inertia, complete rectal mobilization with resection of the lateral rectal ligaments and kinking of a convoluted sigmoid. Hence, the real problem with traditional rectopexy is postoperative constipation, which has dampened the initial expectations driven by the lower recurrence rates associated with the procedure.

11.3.2 Combined Abdominal Rectopexy and Sigmoid Resection

The Frykman-Goldberg procedure [28] is primarily indicated in patients with pre-existing constipation and in those having undergone rectopexy in which the sigmoid colon is so twisted that replacing it in the abdominal cavity would not only be difficult but also would arouse suspicion as to the cause of constipation. For technical reasons, rectopexy is performed after sigmoid resection and without the use of a mesh to minimize the risk of bacterial infection.

The few comparative trials that have been conducted to date (rectopexy alone vs. resection combined with rectopexy) [29–31] have found no meaningful difference in recurrence rates, a lower incidence of postoperative constipation after Frykman-Goldberg procedure (12% vs. 48%), and a statistically significant improvement of incontinence. Enlarging colon resection from sigmoidectomy to left hemicolectomy does not appear to provide additional improvement in bowel function, particularly as regards constipation [32].

Several studies have shown that colon resection with anastomosis increases both the rate of operative mortality (1–2%) and the risk of major complications (34% vs. 22%) [29–31].

11.3.3 Ventral Rectopexy

This procedure derives from the laparotomic technique that Loygue originally devised in 1984 [13]. In 2004, D'Hoore [33] proposed a simplified approach by laparoscopy, in which posterior dissection is limited to exposure of the sacral promontory, opening of the peritoneum to the right of the rectum without resecting the pouch of Douglas, and preparing the anterior rectal subperitoneal fascia as far as the levator muscles. The rectum is then suspended with a mesh (2–3 cm large) fixed cranially to the sacral promontory, and the mesh is then extraperitonealized.

In France, ventral rectopexy is also performed using a more limited dissection, fixation with prosthetic strips, and excision of the lowest portion of the pouch of Douglas [25].

Following initial good outcomes published by D'Hoore's group in Belgium [34] and by others in Great Britain [35, 36], the technique quickly gained wider acceptance owing to its simplicity and effectiveness [37], becoming the abdominal suspension method of choice for prolapse repair. Its indication from FTRP repair was expanded to include rectal intussusception and rectocele, which cause obstructed defecation, and associated with gynecological suspension procedures for the repair of multicompartment prolapses [38].

There is a growing body of evidence documenting good long-term outcomes after ventral rectopexy. Two recent meta-analyses [39, 40] examined the follow-up results in 574 and 789 patients, respectively. The conversion rate was 2.9%; no operative deaths occurred. The postoperative complications rate was lower than 20% and serious complications were noted in 4.8% of patients. The recurrence rate at 2 years was 3.4% and 4.7%, respectively. A net improvement in incontinence was achieved in 30–40% and in up to 80–90% of cases.

Also of interest was the long-term improvement in constipation. Both meta-analyses substantiated the initial reports by D'Hoore [41] and the Oxford group [35]. As compared with traditional rectopexy, a greater improvement in constipation and reduced risk postoperative constipation were associated with ventral rectopexy: improvement in constipation in 3% to over 70% of patients and incidence of new onset constipation or worsening of constipation in 0% to 20% of patients

[39, 40]. The improvement in constipation can be explained by the fact that the lateral rectal ligaments are spared, thus avoiding rectal inertia due to parasympathetic denervation.

Improvement in incontinence (improved in over 80% of patients) has also been reported in elderly patients [42]. Despite advanced age, the basal tone and squeeze pressure values were found to improve during the first 2 months following the operation and continued to improve at 1-year follow-up assessment, with a statistically significant increase in basal tone.

Taken together, these results show that ventral rectopexy is an effective and safe procedure. Although it entails minor and simpler rectal mobilization, it is not associated with a higher recurrence rate. Functional improvement in incontinence and constipation appears promising, making the technique particularly attractive for FTRP repair in older patients [36].

11.3.4 Mesh Selection in Rectopexy Procedures

Following reports of its oncogenicity in experimental studies, use of the Ivalon sponge was abandoned [3]. Most surgeons opted for other types of mesh made from synthetic materials, mostly polypropylene, for traditional rectopexy. Though no significant difference in functional outcome or complication rates has been found for mesh made from absorbable material (polyglycolic acid), it appears to be burdened by a slightly higher rate of recurrence [43].

An emerging problem of synthetic mesh prostheses, sometimes causing severe erosion of rectal or contiguous visceral tissues after ventral rectopexy, has recently come to light. Initially estimated at 1% [44], the risk of erosion seems to be higher (2%) and far greater than that associated with biological prostheses (0.7–2.4% vs. 0–0.7%) [45]. Owing to their antigenic properties, polyester prostheses appear to be more erosive than mesh made from polypropylene or titanium-coated propylene prostheses.

Biological mesh prostheses made from porcine skin or submucosa, though safer, are more expensive. They are less durable, which is thought to be the reason for the higher number of recurrences found at long-term follow-up [46]. Their use in laparoscopic ventral rectopexy should be reserved for young males, women of reproductive age, and particularly for patients at higher risk for developing sepsis due to the presence of comorbid conditions such as diabetes or inflammatory bowel disease, or a history of pelvic radiation therapy or rectal or vaginal surgery [47].

When selecting a synthetic mesh, the material of choice seems to be titanium-coated polypropylene because of its strength and greater resistance to infections [47]. Furthermore, suturing of the mesh to the sacral promontory appears to be safer with staples rather than with simple sutures [48].

11.3.5 Open and Minimally Invasive (Laparoscopy or Robot-Assisted) Procedures

Ventral rectopexy is currently performed in laparoscopy [10, 33, 35, 36].

The wider acceptance of laparoscopic rectopexy has been driven in part by low long-term complications and recurrence rates [27, 39, 49]. Comparative trials evaluating open surgery and laparoscopy have reported no significant differences or even better results in recurrence rates and functional outcomes (improvement in constipation and incontinence) [50, 51]. Moreover, laparoscopy affords the advantages of better cosmesis, less pain, shorter duration of postoperative ileus, and shorter length of hospital stay. Its drawbacks are the longer operative time and limiting problems such as pre-existing abdominal adhesions [10]. Though more expensive than open surgery, the greater cost is offset by shorter hospitalization and less morbidity [30, 50, 51].

Even recent meta-analyses have reported that, in trained hands, long-term recurrence rates and functional outcomes are similar for laparotomy and laparoscopy, while the latter seems to be associated with lower operative complication rates [52, 53].

Robot-assisted surgery appears to combine the advantages of laparoscopy, with better 3D visualization [54–56]. It has been proposed as the technique of choice even in elderly patients [57].

A recent meta-analysis [58] evaluated six studies comparing robotic or laparoscopic ventral rectopexy. There is no statistically significant increase in operating time while there is a shortening in the length of hospital stays. There are no differences in the rate of postoperative complications or conversion rates. However, the question of the benefit-cost ratio with a more expensive method (the robot) remains open.

11.4 Perineal Procedures

11.4.1 Rectosigmoidectomy (Altemeier Procedure)

Perineal resection of the sigmoid colon and rectum for prolapse repair was first described by Auffret in 1882 in France. Following reports by Mikulicz and St. Mark's Hospital in London, the procedure was gradually abandoned because of its high failure rates [59]. It gained renewed interest in the mid twentieth century through refinements by W.A. Altemeier in the United States [60]. According to Altemeier, its combination with levatorplasty was the reason for the less than 3% long-term recurrence rate in his series [61]. The procedure subsequently gained wide acceptance, becoming the most commonly used technique in the United States, particularly in the treatment of high-risk geriatric patients [62]. Many colorectal surgeons now consider it an elective procedure in all patients, irrespective of age [59, 63].

The Altemeier procedure offers distinct advantages for the older patient subpopulation: it can be performed under spinal anesthesia, no scar formation, low postoperative complications, painless rapid course, and early hospital discharge [64].

Controversy mostly surrounds its recurrence rates. In their literature review of studies involving a total of 1635 patients, Cirocco [59] observed a 37% recurrence rate for series treated before 1971 and a 10% rate for series treated after 1971. Specifically regarding geriatric surgery, Altomare et al. [64] examined case series of patients in which the mean age was 77 years (over 80 years in 40% and over 90 years in 7.5% of patients in their own case series) and found a mean recurrence rate of 18%, with a wide individual range (0–58%).

Trials comparing recurrence rates after abdominal procedures (colorectal resection combined with rectopexy) and those after perineal procedures (Altemeier procedure): show that there is no statistically significant difference in the recurrence rate [31, 65]. Moreover, case studies with a follow-up period of up to 4–5 years reported a similar range of recurrence rates, between 0% and 18% [66].

Various reasons have been proposed for the decrease in recurrence rates after Altemeier procedure. Foremost is enhanced awareness of the correct execution of the technique, which entails opening the pouch of Douglas to completely exteriorize the prolapse [59]. Combining the procedure with levatorplasty is also important, as originally suggested by Altemeier [60], and as underlined by some surgeons [67, 68] but not accepted by all [57, 64]. Another explanation for the variability in outcome reported in single case series is the different length of the follow-up, given that the recurrence rate will increase with advancing patient age and that a long term follow-up of elderly patients is difficult to achieve [7, 59, 64]. Other factors (sex, age, length of operative specimen, preoperative incontinence) have not been demonstrated to have a predictive value [64].

The operative mortality rate is extremely low (0.6% of 1635 operations) [59] and the morbidity rate ranges between 3% and 14% [7, 57, 61]. Major early complications (6–7%) include pelvic hematoma, anastomotic dehiscence, sigmoid perforation, and pararectal abscess [64]. The percentage and severity of complications appear to be lower than those associated with abdominal procedures [7, 69, 70].

The use of new technologies (resection with ultrasound or radiofrequency devices and coloanal stapler anastomosis) does not appear to confer meaningful advantages over traditional techniques, except for a lower risk of recurrence (10% vs. 15%) [50].

In most of the patients with pre-existing incontinence, the condition improved: 80–100% in large series [59], and in geriatric patients as well [64]. Particular importance has been given to combining the procedure with levatorplasty to improve postoperative incontinence rather than prevent prolapse recurrence [59, 71, 72].

On the other hand, new onset incontinence was found to develop in 15% of patients who were continent before the operation [59]. This may be explained by the fact that part of the rectal ampulla is removed, resulting in loss of its reservoir function [64]. Comparison between perineal rectosigmoidectomy and an abdominal procedure (resection plus rectopexy) showed that the latter is associated with a significant improvement in continence and less postoperative defecation urgency [65]. For this reason, completing an Altemeier procedure with creation of a pouch has been recommended especially in elderly patients [73].

Postoperative constipation has been reported to improve in 50–60% of cases (range, 15–100%), without worsening of the condition [7, 59, 64]. Therefore, perineal procedures are not burdened by the most severe functional risk associated with rectopexy. The lower risk of postoperative constipation may be attributed to the reduced volume of the rectal ampulla and the consensual resection of the possible intussusception associated with external prolapse.

The good functional outcomes translate into improved quality of life, as measured with the Euro Qol (EQ-5D) questionnaire for measuring generic health status and the Patient Assessment of Constipation Quality of Life (PAC-QoL). The improvement after perineal rectosigmoidectomy, unlike other surgical techniques, does not appear to be influenced by advanced age or comorbidities [74].

11.4.2 Perineal Stapled Prolapse Resection (PSPR)

Scherer [75] recently described a new abdominal perineal resection procedure that offers the advantages of rapidity and ease of execution, which make it of particular interest in geriatric surgery. Based on the variant described by Romano et al. [76], the procedure begins with division of the prolapse using a linear cutter (75 mm) at 3 and 9 o'clock approximately 2 cm above the dentate line. Then resection-suture of the prolapse is performed by a curved cutter stapler (Contour® CCS 30). After insertion, the head is rotated counterclockwise along the two hemi-conferences for complete removal of the prolapse and creation of a suture line cranial to and parallel with the dentate line.

The results are inferior to those obtained with the Altemeier technique, with a recurrence rate of 20% to over 40% in the few cases operated on to date [77, 78]. The reason for such high recurrence may derive from resection performed with traction applied only to the visible portion of the prolapse, resulting in a smaller amount of protruding rectal tissue that can be resected. Furthermore, controlled opening of the pouch of Douglas is not possible, which would allow complete mobilization and exteriorization of the prolapse, and the technique cannot be combined with levatorplasty [79].

Technical limitations may arise from excessive prolapse length (>5–6 cm) and especially excessive prolapse thickness (7–8 mm) owing to the risk of the staples failing to close. Moreover, the method entails performing several steps without visual control: resection-suture of the pouch of Douglas may inadvertently involve the intestinal loops or the vaginal vault in hysterectomized patients. Finally, effective hemostasis cannot be achieved in cases of resection-suturing of a thick mesorectum.

Another problem is the procedure's elevated costs, which may run to about US $1600 if multiple staples are used [79]. This leads to the question of whether the method is justifiable when the Altemeier procedure is less costly and safer in terms of recurrence [59].

Only one recent study [80] compared laparoscopic ventral rectopexy and PSPR in geriatric surgery: the former was found to be better in terms of short-term hospital stays, postoperative complications (7.6% versus 21.3%), long-term functional results and above all recurrence rates (2% versus 20%).

In our opinion, PSPR should be reserved only for high-risk elderly patients (high American Society of Anesthesiologists [ASA] class) in which operative time should be as short as possible and for cases of prolapse repair neither too long nor too thick [81].

11.4.3 Other Perineal Procedures

Encircling holds only a historical interest because of its high failure rates [3].

The Delorme procedure continues to be used in Europe, mainly in France [3, 82]. It may be considered as an alternative to rectosigmoidectomy in cases of short prolapse (<5 cm in length). It is not always easy to perform and it has been associated with recurrence rates of over 30% [83], but lower rates (5–22%) are reported by expert surgeons [77]. The only comparative trial carried out to date [31] found no significant differences in recurrence or functional outcome between the Delorme and the Altemeier procedures. When combined with levatorplasty, the procedure yields improvement in incontinence and recurrence rates, though the difference in recurrence rates was not statistically significant [84].

11.5 Management of Prolapse Recurrence

Most recurrences occur within 3 months of the operation, with the elderly and women at greater risk [85, 86]. The patient's general health condition permitting, recurrent prolapse repair can be performed using the same surgical procedures [87]. While the same access as in the primary operation may be used, most surgeons feel it more prudent in cases of failed rectopexy to switch to a perineal approach. In recurrences after a perineal procedure, especially in elderly patients, the same procedure can be safely and effectively repeated even if laparoscopic ventral rectopexy could be employed if the patient is in good health.

A meta-analysis of studies comparing prolapse recurrence after an abdominal procedure (158 patients) and after a perineal procedure (144 patients) reported a mortality rate of 0% and 15%, respectively; those who had undergone a perineal procedure were evidently in poorer health. The morbidity rate ranged between 0% and 32% and the recurrence rate between 0% and 50% [88]. These results appear somewhat questionable. Undoubtedly, the risk of a new recurrence after repair for prolapse recurrence is higher [85–89].

11.6 Selecting a Surgical Procedure

A long-standing principle that guided the selection of surgical treatment was that abdominal procedures were associated with lower recurrence but greater morbidity, whereas perineal procedures were associated with lower mortality and morbidity and faster postoperative recovery but burdened by higher recurrence [10].

The major factors guiding the choice of treatment in elderly patients are that a perineal procedure can be carried out under spinal anesthesia with shorter operating time, is less demanding on the patient, and allows earlier recovery [10]. Accurate assessment of the patient's general health is essential, given that biological age is more important than chronological age in evaluating elderly patients. Based on the ASA risk classification system, low risk elderly patients may be considered fit for an abdominal procedure, pending a more valid permanent definitive result; whereas a perineal procedure, because it is less demanding on the patient, should be considered for higher risk patients.

Several other factors will also need to be considered when selecting a surgical procedure. An abdominal procedure may be the better choice (combined with a suspension procedure) when repair of multicompartment prolapse (genital or bladder) or co-existing conditions (enterocele or sigmoidocele) needs to be performed in a single stage. In cases of associated gynecological prolapse, priority should be given to repair of the genital prolapse since its treatment (anterior, lateral, posterior colpopexy) may resolve also the posterior problem, obviating the need to operate on the rectum.

On the other hand, because suspending a denervated rectum already weakened due to prolapse may not only be useless but also counterproductive, some surgeons have further expanded the indications for perineal resection [59]. Also, bowel function before surgery may influence the choice of surgical treatment, with the option of selecting between an abdominal or a perineal procedure in patients with normal bowel function. Differently, in patients with pre-existing constipation, owing to the risk of persistent or worsening postoperative constipation, either abdominal rectopexy combined with sigmoid resection or perineal resection, which does not significantly worsen constipation, should be performed [10].

Patient sex is irrelevant in geriatric surgery, whereas in young patients an abdominal procedure can be indicated to reduce the risk of pelvic organ denervation in young males, and mesh suspension in women of reproductive age should be critically considered to minimize the risk of infertility.

11.7 The Evolution of Geriatric Surgery

Historically, patient age has been a major factor in FTRP repair. In the past, perineal procedures, because less demanding on the patient, were the preferred choice in the surgical treatment of elderly patients [66]. Up until 2010, perineal resection was the most commonly performed procedure in patients aged over 70 years in the United States, followed by laparotomy and laparoscopy [90]. Fang et al. [91] retrospectively examined the data from the American College of Surgeons National

Surgical Quality Improvement Program (ACS NSQUIP) database and found that the percentage of patients undergoing an abdominal procedure (by laparotomy or laparoscopy) decreased with advancing patient age. Furthermore, patients aged 80 years or older were twice as likely to undergo a perineal procedure, and those aged under 80 years and with an ASA status of 3 or 4 were 1.5 times more likely than those with an ASA score of 1 or 2.

As the situation continues to evolve, more and more studies are reporting favorably on the wider use of laparoscopic rectopexy in geriatric patients. In patients aged 80 years or older, ventral rectopexy has been associated with a long-term complication rate of 15% and a 3% recurrence rate [36]. A study comparing laparoscopic techniques (rectopexy with or without mesh combined with colon resection) in patients with a mean age of 70 years reported a morbidity rate of 28% and a 3.3% recurrence rate, both of which were similar to those reported for younger patients.

Therefore, it seems that there is a new emerging trend for minimally invasive abdominal rectopexy also in elderly patients, even more than 80 years old [66, 90, 92, 93]. Postoperative mortality and morbidity after ventral rectopexy do not seem to be higher than after perineal surgery, which appear to be burdened by a much higher rate of recurrence. Functional results (improvement of incontinence) would be better, even superior to those of young patients [42].

Therefore, in high volume surgical centers the discriminating factor no longer appears to be the age (old or old old) but only the high ASA score (3–4), with no permissible risks for general anesthesia in abdominal surgery.

Performing a ventral rectopexy in all elderly patients (80 and over 80) appears too radical a suggestion [58].

Once again, the careful assessment of surgical risk and the surgeon's experience appear to be crucial in the choice of the technique. We believe that perineal surgery still plays a fundamental role, especially in high-risk cases, and that abdominal surgery should not be overly chosen in the old and old old patients. More large scale multicenter trials with longer follow-up are still needed.

Acknowledgments The current chapter is an update of the homonymous one, published in the volume Surgical Management of Elderly Patients (Springer, 2018, A. Crucitti ed.) and authored by Francesco Gabrielli, Angelo Guttadauro, Matteo Maternini, and Nicoletta Pecora.

References

1. Kairaluoma MV, Kellokumpu IH. Epidemiologic aspects of complete rectal prolapse. Scand J Surg. 2005;94(3):207–10.
2. Stein EA, Stein DE. Rectal procidentia: diagnosis and management. Gastrointest Endosc Clin N Am. 2006;16(1):189–201.
3. Keighley MRB, Williams NS. Rectal prolapse. In: Keighley MRB, Williams NS, editors. Surgery of the anus rectum and colon. 2nd ed. Saunders; 1999. p. 794–842.
4. Madoff RD, Mellgren A. One hundred years of rectal prolapse surgery. Dis Colon Rectum. 1999;42(4):441–50.
5. Brodén B, Snellman B. Procidentia of the rectum studied with cineradiography. A contribution to the discussion of the causative mechanism. Dis Colon Rectum. 1968;11(5):330–47.

6. Hetzer FH, Senagore A. The evidence for stapled hemorrhoidopexy and STARR. In: Jayne D, Stuto A, editors. Transanal stapling techniques for anorectal prolapse. 1st ed. London: Springer; 2009. p. 95–115.
7. Kim DS, Tsang CB, Wong WD, et al. Complete rectal prolapse: evolution of management and results. Dis Colon Rectum. 1999;42(4):460–6.
8. Khaikin M, Wexner SD. Treatment strategies in obstructed defecation and fecal incontinence. World J Gastroenterol. 2006;12(20):3168–73.
9. Madiba TE, Baig MK, Wexner SD. Surgical management of rectal prolapse. Arch Surg. 2005;140(1):63–73.
10. Tou S, Brown SR, Nelson RL. Surgery for complete (full-thickness) rectal prolapse in adults. Cochrane Database Syst Rev. 2015;2015(11):CD001758.
11. Karas JR, Uranues S, Altomare DF, et al. No rectopexy versus rectopexy following rectal mobilization for full-thickness rectal prolapse: a randomized controlled trial. Dis Colon Rectum. 2011;54(1):29–34.
12. Wells C. New operation for rectal prolapse. Proc R Soc Med. 1959;52(8):602–3.
13. Loygue J, Huguier M, Malafosse M, Biotois H. Complete prolapse of the rectum. A report on 140 cases treated by rectopexy. Br J Surg. 1971;58(11):847–8.
14. Ripstein CB. Procidentia: definitive corrective surgery. Dis Colon Rectum. 1972;15(5):334–6.
15. Novell JR, Osborne MJ, Winslet MC, Lewis AA. Prospective randomized trial of Ivalon sponge versus sutured rectopexy for full-thickness rectal prolapse. Br J Surg. 1994;81(6):904–6.
16. Speakman CTM, Madden MV, Nicholls RJ, Kamm MA. Lateral ligament division during rectopexy causes constipation but prevents recurrence: results of a prospective randomized study. Br J Surg. 1991;78(12):1431–3.
17. Selvaggi F, Scotto di Carlo E, Silvestri L, et al. Surgical treatment of rectal prolapse: a randomised study. Br J Surg. 1993;80(Suppl):S89.
18. Mollen RM, Kuijpers JH, van Hoek F. Effects of rectal mobilization and lateral ligaments division on colonic and anorectal function. Dis Colon Rectum. 2000;43(9):1283–7.
19. Watts JD, Rothenberger DA, Buls JG, et al. The management of procidentia. 30 years' experience. Dis Colon Rectum. 1985;28(2):96–102.
20. Madbouly KM, Senagore AJ, Delaney CP, et al. Clinically based management of rectal prolapse. Surg Endosc. 2003;17(1):99–103.
21. Raftopoulos Y, Senagore AJ, Di Giuro G, et al. Recurrence rates after abdominal surgery for complete rectal prolapse: a multicenter pooled analysis of 643 individual patient data. Dis Colon Rectum. 2005;48(6):1200–6.
22. Portier G, Iovino F, Lazorthes F. Surgery for rectal prolapse: Orr-Loygue ventral rectopexy with limited dissection prevents postoperative-induced constipation without increasing recurrence. Dis Colon Rectum. 2006;49(8):1136–40.
23. Gabrielli F, Campanelli GP, Leopaldi E, et al. Terapia chirurgica del prolasso rettale: vantaggi e limiti delle rettopessie per via addominale. Chirurgia. 1993;6:535–40.
24. Lechaux JP, Atienza P, Goasguen N, et al. Prosthetic rectopexy to the pelvic floor and sigmoidectomy for rectal prolapse. Am J Surg. 2001;182(5):465–9.
25. Laubert T, Kleemann M, Schorcht A, et al. Laparoscopic resection rectopexy for rectal prolapse: a single-center study during 16 years. Surg Endosc. 2010;24(10):2401–6.
26. Dulucq JL, Wintringer P, Mahajna A. Clinical and functional outcome of laparoscopic posterior rectopexy (Wells) for full-thickness rectal prolapse. A prospective study. Surg Endosc. 2007;21(12):2226–30.
27. Lechaux D, Trebuchet G, Siproudhis L, Campion JP. Laparoscopic rectopexy for full-thickness rectal prolapse: a single-institution retrospective study evaluating surgical outcome. Surg Endosc. 2005;19(4):514–8.
28. Frykman HM, Goldberg SM. The surgical treatment of rectal procidentia. Surg Gynecol Obstet. 1969;129(6):1225–30.
29. Luukkonen P, Mikkonen U, Järvinen H. Abdominal rectopexy with sigmoidectomy versus rectopexy alone for rectal prolapse: a prospective, randomized study. Int J Color Dis. 1992;7(4):219–22.

30. Tjandra JJ, Fazio VW, Church JM, et al. Ripstein procedure is an effective treatment for rectal prolapse without constipation. Dis Colon Rectum. 1993;36(5):501–7.
31. Senapati A, Gray RG, Middleton LJ, et al. PROSPER: a randomised comparison of surgical treatments for rectal prolapse. Color Dis. 2013;15(7):858–68.
32. Yoshioka K, Heyen F, Keighley MRB. Functional results after posterior abdominal rectopexy for rectal prolapse. Dis Colon Rectum. 1989;32(10):835–8.
33. D'Hoore A, Cadoni R, Penninckx F. Long-term outcome of laparoscopic ventral rectopexy for total rectal prolapse. Br J Surg. 2004;91(11):1500–5.
34. D'Hoore A, Penninckx F. Laparoscopic ventral recto(colpo)pexy for rectal prolapse: surgical technique and outcome for 109 patients. Surg Endosc. 2006;20(12):1919–23.
35. Boons P, Collinson R, Cunningham C, Lindsey I. Laparoscopic ventral rectopexy for external rectal prolapse improves constipation and avoids de novo constipation. Color Dis. 2010;12(6):526–32.
36. Wijffels N, Cunningham C, Dixon A, et al. Laparoscopic ventral rectopexy for external rectal prolapse is safe and effective in the elderly. Does this make perineal procedures obsolete? Color Dis. 2011;13(5):561–6.
37. Auguste T, Dubreuil A, Bost R, et al. Technical and functional results after laparoscopic rectopexy to the promontory for complete rectal prolapse. Prospective study in 54 consecutive patients. Gastroenterol Clin Biol. 2006;30(5):659–63.
38. Gurland B. Ventral mesh rectopexy: is this the new standard for surgical treatment of pelvic organ prolapse? Dis Colon Rectum. 2014;57(12):1446–7.
39. Faucheron JL, Trilling B, Girard E, et al. Anterior rectopexy for full-thickness rectal prolapse: technical and functional results. World J Gastroenterol. 2015;21(16):5049–55.
40. Samaranayake CB, Luo C, Plank AW, et al. Systematic review on ventral rectopexy for rectal prolapse and intussusception. Color Dis. 2010;12(6):504–12.
41. van Geluwe B, Wolthuis A, Penninckx F, D'Hoore A. Lessons learned after more than 400 laparoscopic ventral rectopexies. Acta Chir Belg. 2013;113(2):103–6.
42. Bjerke T, Mynster T. Laparoscopic ventral rectopexy in an elderly population with external rectal prolapse: clinical and anal manometric results. Int J Color Dis. 2014;29(10):1257–62.
43. Galili Y, Rabau M. Comparison of polyglycolic acid and polypropylene mesh for rectopexy in the treatment of rectal prolapse. Eur J Surg. 1997;163(6):445–8.
44. Smart NJ, Pathak S, Boorman P, Daniels IR. Synthetic or biological mesh use in laparoscopic ventral mesh rectopexy: a systematic review. Color Dis. 2013;15(6):650–4.
45. Evans C, Stevenson AR, Sileri P, et al. A multicenter collaboration to assess the safety of laparoscopic ventral rectopexy. Dis Colon Rectum. 2015;58(8):799–807.
46. Bhandarkar DS. Laparoscopic rectopexy for complete rectal prolapse: mesh, no mesh or a ventral mesh? J Minim Access Surg. 2014;10(1):1–3.
47. Mercer-Jones MA, D'Hoore A, Dixon AR, et al. Consensus on ventral rectopexy: report of a panel of experts. Color Dis. 2014;16(2):82–8.
48. Darzi A, Henry MM, Guillou PJ, et al. Stapled laparoscopic rectopexy for rectal prolapse. Surg Endosc. 1995;9(3):301–3.
49. Kariv Y, Delaney CP, Casillas S, et al. Long-term outcome after laparoscopic and open surgery for rectal prolapse: a case-control study. Surg Endosc. 2006;20(1):35–42.
50. Boccasanta P, Venturi M, Barbieri S, Roviaro G. Impact of new technologies on the clinical and functional outcome of Altemeier's procedure: a randomized, controlled trial. Dis Colon Rectum. 2006;49(5):652–60.
51. Salkeld G, Bagia M, Solomon M. Economic impact of laparoscopic versus open abdominal rectopexy. Br J Surg. 2004;91(9):1188–91.
52. Purkayastha S, Tekkis P, Athanasiou T, et al. A comparison of open vs. laparoscopic abdominal rectopexy for full-thickness rectal prolapse: a meta-analysis. Dis Colon Rectum. 2005;48(10):1930–40.
53. Sajid MS, Siddiqui MR, Baig MK. Open vs laparoscopic repair of full-thickness rectal prolapse: a re-meta-analysis. Color Dis. 2010;12(6):515–25.

54. Munz Y, Moorthy K, Kudchadkar R, et al. Robotic assisted rectopexy. Am J Surg. 2004;187(1):88–92.
55. Heemskerk J, de Hoog DENM, van Gemert WG, et al. Robot-assisted vs. conventional laparoscopic rectopexy for rectal prolapse: a comparative study on costs and time. Dis Colon Rectum. 2007;50(11):1825–30.
56. Mäkelä-Kaikkonen J, Rautio T, Klintrup K, et al. Robotic-assisted and laparoscopic ventral rectopexy in the treatment of rectal prolapse: a matched-pairs study of operative details and complications. Tech Coloproctol. 2014;18(2):151–5.
57. Flynn J, Larach JT, Kong JCH, et al. Robotic versus laparoscopic ventral mesh rectopexy: a systematic review and meta-analysis. Int J Color Dis. 2021;36(8):1621–31.
58. Ergüder E, Verkade C, Wasowicz DK, et al. Laparoscopic ventral mesh rectopexy in the oldest old is safe: the race is run. Tech Coloproctol. 2024;28(1):46.
59. Cirocco WC. The Altemeier procedure for rectal prolapse: an operation for all ages. Dis Colon Rectum. 2010;53(12):1618–23.
60. Altemeier WA, Giuseffi J, Hoxworth P. Treatment of extensive prolapse of the rectum in aged or debilitated patients. Arch Surg. 1952;65(1):72–80.
61. Altemeier WA, Culbertson WR, Schowengerdt C, Hunt J. Nineteen years' experience with the one-stage perineal repair of rectal prolapse. Ann Surg. 1971;173(6):993–1006.
62. Schoetz DJ Jr. Evolving practice patterns in colon and rectal surgery. J Am Coll Surg. 2006;203(3):322–7.
63. Glasgow SC, Birnbaum EH, Kodner IJ, et al. Recurrence and quality of life following perineal proctectomy for rectal prolapse. J Gastrointest Surg. 2008;12(8):1446–51.
64. Altomare DF, Binda G, Ganio E, et al. Long-term outcome of Altemeier's procedure for rectal prolapse. Dis Colon Rectum. 2009;52(4):698–703.
65. Deen KI, Grant E, Billingham C, Keighley MR. Abdominal resection rectopexy with pelvic floor repair versus perineal rectosigmoidectomy and pelvic floor repair for full-thickness rectal prolapse. Br J Surg. 1994;81(2):302–4.
66. Hrabe J, Gurland B. Optimizing treatment for rectal prolapse. Clin Colon Rectal Surg. 2016;29(3):271–6.
67. Agachan F, Pfeiffer J, Joo JS, et al. Results of perineal procedures for the treatment of rectal prolapse. Am Surg. 1997;63(1):9–12.
68. Williams JG, Rothenberger DA, Madoff RD, Goldberg SM. Treatment of rectal prolapse in the elderly by perineal rectosigmoidectomy. Dis Colon Rectum. 1992;35(9):830–4.
69. Azimuddin K, Khubchandani IT, Rosen L, et al. Rectal prolapse: a search for the "best" operation. Am Surg. 2001;67(7):622–7.
70. Habr-Gama A, Jacob CE, Jorge JM, et al. Rectal procidentia treatment by perineal rectosigmoidectomy combined with levator ani repair. Hepato-Gastroenterology. 2006;53(68):213–7.
71. Chun SW, Pikarsky AJ, You SY, et al. Perineal rectosigmoidectomy for rectal prolapse: role of levatorplasty. Tech Coloproctol. 2004;8(1):3–8.
72. Prasad ML, Pearl RK, Abcarian H, et al. Perineal proctectomy, posterior rectopexy, and postanal levator repair for the treatment of rectal prolapse. Dis Colon Rectum. 1986;29(9):547–52.
73. Yoshioka K, Ogunbiyi OA, Keighley MRB. Pouch perineal rectosigmoidectomy gives better functional results than conventional rectosigmoidectomy in elderly patients with rectal prolapse. Br J Surg. 1998;85(11):1525–6.
74. Kim M, Reibetanz J, Schlegel N, et al. Perineal rectosigmoidectomy: quality of life. Color Dis. 2013;15(8):1000–6.
75. Scherer R, Marti L, Hetzer F. Perineal stapled prolapse resection: a new procedure for external rectal prolapse. Dis Colon Rectum. 2008;51(11):1727–30.
76. Romano G, Bianco F, Caggiano L. Modified perineal stapled rectal resection with contour transtar for full-thickness rectal prolapse. Color Dis. 2009;11(8):878–81.
77. Tschuor C, Limani P, Nocito A, et al. Perineal stapled prolapse resection for external rectal prolapse: is it worthwhile in the long-term? Tech Coloproctol. 2013;17(5):537–40.
78. Raahave D, Jensen AK, Dammegaard L, Pedersen IK. Primary and repeated perineal stapled prolapse resection. Tech Coloproctol. 2016;20(12):853–7.

79. Ram E, Krissi H, Zbar A, et al. Perineal stapled prolapse resection (PSPR) in elderly patients for external rectal prolapse: early experience. Tech Coloproctol. 2014;18(11):1003–7.
80. Habeeb TAAM, Podda M, Chiaretti M, et al. Comparative study of laparoscopic ventral mesh rectopexy versus perineal stapler resection for external full-thickness rectal prolapse in elderly patients: enhanced outcomes and reduced recurrence rates - a retrospective cohort study. Tech Coloproctol. 2024;28(1):48.
81. Maternini M, Guttadauro A, Pecora N, Gabrielli F. Perineal stapled prolapse resection (PSPR) for external rectal prolapse in high morbidity patients. Ann Ital Chir. 2016;87:476–80.
82. Tsunoda A, Yasuda N, Yokoyama N, et al. Delorme's procedure for rectal prolapse. Clinical and physiological analysis. Dis Colon Rectum. 2003;46(9):1260–5.
83. Senapati A, Nicholls RJ, Thomson JP, Phillips RK. Results of Delorme's procedure for rectal prolapse. Dis Colon Rectum. 1994;37(5):456–60.
84. Youssef M, Thabet W, El Nakeeb A, et al. Comparative study between Delorme operation with or without postanal repair and levateroplasty in treatment of complete rectal prolapse. Int J Surg. 2013;11(1):52–8.
85. Hool GR, Hull TL, Fazio VW. Surgical treatment of recurrent complete rectal prolapse: a thirty-year experience. Dis Colon Rectum. 1997;40(3):270–2.
86. Pikarsky AJ, Joo JS, Wexner SD, et al. Recurrent rectal prolapse: what is the next good option? Dis Colon Rectum. 2000;43(9):1273–6.
87. Steele SR, Goetz LH, Minami S, et al. Management of recurrent rectal prolapse: surgical approach influences outcome. Dis Colon Rectum. 2006;49(4):440–5.
88. Hotouras A, Ribas Y, Zakeri S, et al. A systematic review of the literature on the surgical management of recurrent rectal prolapse. Color Dis. 2015;17(8):657–64.
89. Ding JH, Canedo J, Lee SH, et al. Perineal rectosigmoidectomy for primary and recurrent rectal prolapse: are the results comparable the second time? Dis Colon Rectum. 2012;55(6):666–70.
90. Clark CE 3rd, Jupiter DC, Thomas JS, Papaconstantinou HT. Rectal prolapse in the elderly: trends in surgical management and outcomes from the American College of Surgeons National Surgical Quality Improvement Program database. J Am Coll Surg. 2012;215(5):709–14.
91. Fang SH, Cromwell JW, Wilkins KB, et al. Is the abdominal repair of rectal prolapse safer then perineal repair in the highest risk patients? An NSQIP analysis. Dis Colon Rectum. 2012;55(11):1167–72.
92. De Carlo G, Belkovsky M, Ban KA, et al. Management of rectal prolapse in octogenarians: lesson learned in 13 years' experience from a high-volume center. Updat Surg. 2025;77(8):2417–24.
93. Gültekin FA, Wong MTC, Podevin J, et al. Safety of laparoscopic ventral rectopexy in the elderly: results from a nationwide database. Dis Colon Rectum. 2015;58(3):339–43.

12 Emergency General Surgery in the Elderly

Luca Ansaloni, Federico Coccolini, and Fausto Catena

12.1 Introduction to Emergency General Surgery

Emergency general surgery (EGS) is vital for preventing death or long-term impairment in patients with critical issues like hemorrhage or trauma. Quick intervention greatly affects outcomes. Elderly patients face higher risks due to age and comorbidities complicating surgical decisions. However, age should not exclude them from essential surgery [1–3].

12.2 Demographics of the Elderly Population in Emergency General Surgery

Population aging presents challenges, with over 20% of Europeans being over 65, an age group that utilizes healthcare resources three times more than those under 66. Limited specialized services worsen outcomes. An increase in patients aged over 80 needing emergency surgeries complicates care owing to pre-existing conditions that demand ongoing post-admission healthcare. The effective use of acute-care beds is crucial, making frailty assessment during emergencies challenging, and tools like the American Society of Anesthesiologists (ASA) score aid in risk stratification. Adapting to demographic changes is essential for healthcare systems addressing elderly patients' emergency surgical care needs [1, 3, 4].

L. Ansaloni (✉)
Department of Emergency Surgery, Fondazione IRCSS Policlinico San Matteo, Pavia, Italy
e-mail: l.ansaloni@smatteo.pv.it

F. Coccolini
Department of Emergency Surgery, Pisa University Hospital, Pisa, Italy

F. Catena
Department of Medical and Surgical Sciences, Alma Mater Studiorum University of Bologna, Bologna, Italy

P. Carcoforo, F. Catena (eds.), *Geriatric Surgery*, Updates in Surgery,
https://doi.org/10.1007/978-3-032-24281-5_12

12.3 Common Surgical Emergencies in the Elderly

EGS in the elderly presents significant challenges for surgeons and patients due to limited clinical history and urgent care needs, increasing morbidity and mortality risks. With the aging population, especially in high-income countries where those aged over 60 may reach 20% and those over 80, 6% by 2050, emergency surgeries are expected to rise. Currently, 30% of 32 million surgeries annually are emergencies, with 50% of 4 million U.S. surgeries involving patients aged 65 and older, stressing healthcare systems and requiring specialized training [1, 5].

12.3.1 Appendicitis

The SIFIPAC/WSES/SICG/SIMEU clinical guidelines established jointly by the Italian Society of Surgical Pathophysiology, Italian Society of Geriatric Surgery, World Society of Emergency Surgery, Italian Society of Emergency Medicine in 2019 indicate that the incidence of acute appendicitis decreases with age, with only 15% of patients over 50 being affected compared to nearly 30% of younger individuals. Elderly patients face higher mortality rates, intensified over 5 years, while younger groups show rates of 0–1%. The risk of complicated appendicitis increases in older patients, with 1–80% experiencing perforation or abscess versus 3–29% in those under 50. Contributing factors include vascular issues, late diagnosis, and protracted hospital stays resulting in poorer postoperative outcomes. Appendectomy mortality rates rise significantly with age, exceeding 1% in nonagenarians. Controversy exists over the best surgical approach for older adults, as appendicitis is rare in this demographic, constituting only 5–10% of cases and necessitating consideration of atypical causes such as cancer [6–8].

12.3.2 Cholecystitis

Cholecystitis largely arises from gallstone disease, impacting 10–15% of surgical patients with acute cases. It often requires urgent surgery, like cholecystectomy, which can be laparoscopic or open. Perioperative mortality is generally below 1%, but increases to 6% in the elderly. Implementing Enhanced Recovery After Surgery (ERAS®) principles may improve outcomes, particularly for older patients, by enhancing recovery through strategies like carbohydrate loading, fluid management, early feeding, and mobilization [9].

12.3.3 Diverticulitis

Diverticulitis is common among the elderly especially in Western countries, and involves inflammation of colonic diverticula that can lead to serious infections. Approximately 25% of those with diverticular disease may develop diverticulitis, with severe complications like perforation and peritonitis often requiring emergency surgery. Timely surgical intervention is essential for purulent or fecaloid perforated diverticulitis to prevent further complications. Delays worsen outcomes for elderly patients. The initial focus is on hemodynamic optimization, including fluid resuscitation and vasoactive agents, followed by appropriate surgical procedures based on stability. Hartmann's procedure is still typical for stable patients, though recent studies advocate for primary resection with anastomosis to lower mortality and complications when feasible [10, 11].

12.3.4 Bowel Obstruction

Bowel obstruction is a serious issue, especially in the elderly, accounting for 6–20% of emergency surgeries. It can be categorized by cause, gastrointestinal location, and severity. In older adults, around 80% of obstructions are due to adhesions, hernias, and tumors, with small bowel obstructions being most common. Mechanical obstructions hinder normal bowel function, leading to distension and fluid buildup. While some cases can be managed conservatively, others require a multidisciplinary approach for comprehensive care. Gastrografin may be an effective treatment for certain bowel obstructions, improving bowel activity and helping content passage [12].

12.3.5 Peptic Ulcer

Peptic ulcers, caused by inflammation of the gastroduodenal mucosa are common in the elderly, and present with acute abdominal pain and vomiting. Complicated cases require emergency surgery, with techniques depending on the ulcer's specifics and location. Treatments may involve omental patch closure or resection with drainage. Perforation poses serious risks for older patients, especially those with steroid or NSAID use and late diagnoses, which can lead to peritonitis or sepsis. While simple closure suffices for many duodenal ulcers, gastric ulcers often require resection. Surgical risks are higher in older patients, and mortality from hemorrhage surpasses that of perforation, making surgery a last resort [13–15].

12.3.6 Polytrauma

Multiple trauma is the fourth leading cause of emergency evaluations in the elderly, especially those over 75. Most injuries affect the extremities, and elderly individuals have a 50% higher rate of emergency admissions than younger people. Severe injuries do not always lead to higher 30-day mortality, but elderly men over 70 with severe brain injuries have significantly increased mortality rates. Timely and tailored treatment is crucial to minimize risks [16, 17].

12.4 Preoperative Assessment

A thorough preoperative assessment of elderly patients undergoing EGS is critical to reduce complications and mortality. These patients typically present multiple comorbidities and medications that complicate care. A comprehensive evaluation ensures safety by assessing health risks and identifying necessary treatments or consultations. It also addresses social factors like postoperative care, which is essential as elderly individuals often require additional rehabilitation and skilled nursing. In emergencies, these patients frequently arrive in a compromised state, making an in-depth review of medical history, physical exams, and diagnostic tests essential [18–20].

12.4.1 Risk Stratification

Risk stratification in elderly emergency surgery patients is crucial for assessing operative risk and physiologic reserve. The ASA classification ranges from optimal health (ASA 1) to brain-dead (ASA 6), with an "E" suffix for emergencies, resulting in ASA 1E to ASA 5E. Most elderly patients undergoing urgent abdominal surgery are typically classified as ASA 2E to 5E, denoting significant physiologic instability. This classification predicts operative mortality and complications better than age or comorbidities. While no universal risk assessment method exists, eight variables are essential for stratification: severity of health condition, reason for surgery, procedure complexity, emergency status, surgery timeframe, patient age and reserve, choice of anesthetic, and complication potential. Identifying high-risk patients aids resource allocation, consent, and postoperative planning [20, 21].

12.4.2 Comorbidities

Older patients have a higher mortality risk after emergency surgeries, with preoperative comorbidities being more important than the emergencies themselves. Elective surgeries, as for incarcerated hernias, can decrease morbidity and mortality. Most individuals over 80 have multiple comorbidities and face daily living challenges. Over 60% need extra healthcare after admission, yet long-term survival rates are good, with half surviving 3 years after surgery. As life expectancy increases, demand for acute care services will rise. Emergency surgeries in the elderly carry significant risks tied to comorbid conditions. The Charlson Comorbidity Index can aid in selecting candidates for elective procedures. High-comorbidity patients often face worse outcomes, emphasizing the need for specialized geriatric care, which has been shown to lower mortality rates [20, 21].

12.4.3 Functional Status Evaluation

Assessing health status is crucial for preoperative evaluation. A thorough assessment—with physical examinations, medical history, and laboratory tests—helps the perioperative team gauge the risks and enhance health before surgery. This is especially vital for the elderly, who need detailed medical histories and functional status assessments. The Duke Activity Status Index (DASI) measures functional capacity in metabolic equivalents (METs), where activities requiring 4 METs include walking 3–4 mph or light housework. Functional capacity below 4 METs indicates higher cardiac risk, postoperative mortality, and may point to frailty impacting future geriatric care [18].

12.5 Anesthesia Considerations

Choice of anesthesia depends on the procedure and patient health. Regional anesthesia is safer for elderly patients owing to lower risks of respiratory failure and confusion; general anesthesia poses higher risks in emergencies. Customized plans for frail patients with organ issues should prioritize simplicity and minimal invasiveness. A combination of regional and low-dose intravenous anesthesia is ideal. Inhalational anesthesia may help transition to total intravenous anesthesia, but precautions against hypoxemia and hypotension are crucial. Postoperative delirium, tied to neuroinflammation, necessitates vital sign monitoring and effective pain management in the post-anesthesia care unit to prevent cardiovascular complications [22, 23].

12.5.1 Types of Anesthesia

Emergency surgery in older patients presents challenges for surgical teams. Factors like choice of anesthesia, preoperative assessments, and minimization of complications require consideration of differences between older and younger patients. Regional anesthesia may reduce pulmonary issues, while general anesthesia can decrease functional capacity and exacerbate oxygen disparities, worsening chronic respiratory conditions and postoperative complications [23–25].

12.5.2 Anesthesia Risks in the Elderly

Elderly patients face higher risks of impaired recovery and complications after surgery with general anesthesia. They exhibit lower recovery scores and psychomotor function, with 10% having extended post-anesthesia care unit stays, particularly those with delirium. Intensive care unit admissions are common, and frail elderly patients have less than 60% 30-day survival rates. Organ changes with aging necessitate careful maintenance of perfusion. Regional anesthesia is safer, lowering stress responses and thromboembolic risks while providing effective pain relief [23, 26].

12.6 Postoperative Care

Frail patients facing emergency surgery are at a higher risk of poor postoperative outcomes, with challenges in pain management and recognition of complications affecting their recovery. Effective pain control is essential and based on clinical and mechanical strategies. Monitoring complications such as myocardial infarction, stroke, pneumonia, and renal failure is crucial, necessitating a multidisciplinary team including surgeons, geriatricians, and healthcare personnel. Early geriatric consultation can notably decrease mortality, particularly in elderly patients with emergency hip fractures [27].

12.6.1 Pain Management

Postoperative pain management is a critical consideration for elderly patients undergoing EGS. Adequate assessment and management of pain are vital for successful recovery in this population. Inadequate pain relief can result in lasting disability and a compromised quality of life. Additionally, insufficient analgesia can elicit detrimental stress responses, including tachycardia and immune system dysfunction, during the perioperative period [28, 29].

12.6.2 Complications and Monitoring

Complications can arise from diseases or treatments, necessitating prompt intervention for issues like hemorrhage, perforation, and thrombosis. Elderly patients face elevated risks and require close monitoring due to their altered responses to inflammation, making them more prone to severe infections such as sepsis. Symptoms can be vague, and even minimal signs of peritonitis call for swift laparotomy. Quick corrections are vital for cardiac rhythm disturbances and drug interactions. Additionally, anesthesia and analgesics can exacerbate pulmonary issues, while sedation and delirium can complicate emergency management [30].

12.7 Ethical Considerations

Informed consent and end-of-life decisions pose challenges in emergency surgery for the elderly. With high death risk and limited long-term survival, ethical dilemmas arise. Developing an ethical framework based on studies can guide clinicians, patients, and families in decision-making [1].

12.7.1 Informed Consent

Informed consent for elderly patients in EGS is crucial, as procedures aim to prevent death or serious complications. The process must be swift, considering limited decision-making time and specific clinical factors like comorbidities and cognitive issues in older patients. Balancing surgical urgency with clear communication about risks, benefits and alternatives is vital, ensuring the patient or their representative is well informed despite time constraints [13].

12.7.2 End-of-Life Decisions

End-of-life decisions after emergency surgery in the elderly pose significant challenges, often made during acute health crises in hospitals lacking adequate palliative care. The emphasis should transition from aggressive interventions to symptom management and stabilization. Improved shared decision-making and coordination with palliative care can assist patients and families during these critical choices [1].

12.8 Multidisciplinary Approach to Care

Emergency surgical care is placed at the interface where the stress of comorbid physiological conditions meets an unpredictable and often adverse and time-sensitive surgical pathology. In the elderly, this interplay is substantially aggravated, and reliance on experienced surgeons, a good multidisciplinary team, and adherence to the principles of a radical treatment approach are paramount if outcomes are to be improved [1]. Postoperative protocols specifically developed to address the needs of older adults can improve outcomes, but standardized protocols have not yet been developed [27].

12.8.1 Role of Geriatricians

The rising number of elderly patients needing emergency surgery has led to specialists focused on their surgical care. These specialists understand the conditions requiring urgent treatment and the physiological changes of aging. Such knowledge is vital for optimal care. Comprehensive assessment and patient-centered interventions, including discharge planning, enhance outcomes for older emergency patients [31].

12.8.2 Role of Nurses

Nursing care is essential for successful emergency surgery in the elderly, and it involves a variety of advanced skills throughout all phases, from assessment to postoperative care [30, 32]. Postoperative admission to a geriatric unit lowers mortality, while geriatric consultation teams improve clinical outcomes. Skilled nursing care is essential for wound management and adjusting to psychological, social, and functional recovery changes. Elderly patients undergoing EGS require teamwork involving surgeons, anesthetists, and nurses for improved outcomes and reduced complications [12].

12.9 Impact of Emergency Surgery on Quality of Life

The loss of independence and return to baseline after emergency surgery impact on patient's consent for life-saving procedures. Understanding futility is crucial in decision-making, as the criteria for intervention versus non-intervention remain unclear. Factors include postoperative quality of life, complications, and regaining functional status. High-quality research is essential to assess emergency surgery's impact on elderly patients, assisting the multidisciplinary team in consent discussions [3].

12.10 Long-Term Outcomes Post-Surgery

Limited information on long-term outcomes after emergency surgery in the elderly shows decent survival rates at 1, 2, and 3 years, but many deaths are not due to surgery. Over 60% of patients need extra support, such as rehabilitation or nursing homes, leading to a decline in functional quality of life. While they may survive, elderly patients often experience poor postoperative quality of life and face unfavorable outcomes compared to younger patients [7, 32, 33].

12.11 Futility in Geriatric Emergency Surgery

The concept of futility in EGS for elderly patients presents significant challenges due to heightened risks, including complications, loss of autonomy, and increased mortality. The hazards of surgery grow with age, irrespective of the acute conditions involved. Older adults undergoing emergency surgery face higher mortality rates than those undergoing elective surgeries, making it difficult for clinicians to decide on major surgical interventions in patients with limited life expectancy and multiple health issues [21, 34].

12.12 Future Directions in Elderly Surgical Care

As the elderly population grows, EGS is on the rise, necessitating improved data sharing and patient education for better results. Preventing complications like delirium and pneumonia is crucial for recovery. Geriatric surgical care should incorporate a multidisciplinary approach using techniques such as laparoscopic interventions and thorough pre- and postoperative protocols to address age-related health issues. Innovation in EGS is essential to tackle the challenges faced by elderly patients, who often have limited physiological reserves and multiple comorbidities. Mortality rates vary from 0% to 30%, even with advancements in elective surgery. Serious postoperative complications can delay recovery and increase nursing care costs. Research into outpatient emergency surgery may decrease lengthy hospital stays, though its effects on older adults require further study. Understanding the impact of frailty on surgical risk is vital, as many elderly individuals find it hard to regain full function after surgery, highlighting the need for targeted research to enhance recovery in this vulnerable population [5, 7, 12, 35].

12.13 Conclusion

Implementing new diagnostic and treatment strategies could improve outcomes for elderly emergency surgery patients. Postoperative care must be tailored to the specific reason for surgery. Managing sepsis and frailty is as crucial as resuscitation and open abdomen care. Ethical decisions in emergencies can be supported by routinely checking advance directives and care planning. The surgical approach should follow principles of damage control and integration of evidence-based quality measures. A minimum set of quality indicators include sepsis control, maintaining normothermia, appropriate antimicrobial therapy, lung protective ventilation, and enhanced recovery protocols based on avoidance of perioperative fluid excess and opioids, and functional patient mobilization. Patients with a high burden of comorbidity/advanced stage of disease and futile prognosis should be identified early and either managed nonoperatively or referred for palliative care [36, 37].

References

1. Søreide K, Desserud KF. Emergency surgery in the elderly: the balance between function, frailty, fatality and futility. Scand J Trauma Resusc Emerg Med. 2015;23:10.
2. Limmer S, Unger L, Czymek R, et al. Emergency thoracic surgery in elderly patients. JRSM Short Rep. 2011;2(2):13.
3. Merani S, Payne J, Padwal RS, et al. Predictors of in-hospital mortality and complications in very elderly patients undergoing emergency surgery. World J Emerg Surg. 2014;9:43.
4. Abdul Rahim K, Shaikh NQ, Lakhdir MPA, et al. No healthcare coverage, big problem: lack of insurance for older population associated with worse emergency general surgery outcomes. Trauma Surg Acute Care Open. 2024;9(1):e001165.
5. Michalik M, Dowgiałło-Wnukiewicz N, Lech P, Zacharz K. Surgery of the elderly in emergency room mode. Is there a place for laparoscopy? Wideochir Inne Tech Maloinwazyjne. 2017;12(2):115–9.
6. Fugazzola P, Ceresoli M, Agnoletti V, et al. The SIFIPAC/WSES/SICG/SIMEU guidelines for diagnosis and treatment of acute appendicitis in the elderly (2019 edition). World J Emerg Surg. 2020;15(1):19.

7. Wang D, Dong T, Shao Y, et al. Laparoscopy versus open appendectomy for elderly patients, a meta-analysis and systematic review. BMC Surg. 2019;19(1):54.
8. Das R, Cantor JP, Vu TQ. Two concurrent appendiceal neoplasms in an elderly patient: a case report. Int J Surg Case Rep. 2017;40:124–6.
9. Wiggins T, Markar SR, Mackenzie H, et al. Evolution in the management of acute cholecystitis in the elderly: population-based cohort study. Surg Endosc. 2018;32(10):4078–86.
10. Cirocchi R, Sapienza P, Anania G, et al. State-of-the-art surgery for sigmoid diverticulitis. Langenbeck's Arch Surg. 2022;407(1):1–14.
11. Bordeianou L, Hodin R. Controversies in the surgical management of sigmoid diverticulitis. J Gastrointest Surg. 2007;11(4):542–8.
12. Ozturk E, van Iersel M, Stommel MM, et al. Small bowel obstruction in the elderly: a plea for comprehensive acute geriatric care. World J Emerg Surg. 2018;13:48.
13. Idris M, Smiley A, Patel S, Latifi R. Risk factors for mortality in emergently admitted patients with acute gastric ulcer: an analysis of 15,538 patients in national inpatient sample, 2005-2014. Int J Environ Res Public Health. 2022;19(23):16263.
14. Abdalgalil HH, Ismail AS, Alshmaily HO, Alshammari DS. A conservative management of perforated peptic ulcer: a case report. Cureus. 2024;16(3):e56491.
15. Rigopoulos A, Ramboiu S, Georgescu I. A critical evaluation of surgical treatment of perforated ulcer. Curr Health Sci J. 2011;37(2):75–8.
16. Abhilash KPP, Pradeeptha S, Cris A, et al. Severe or not so severe? The gravity of geriatric trauma. J Family Med Prim Care. 2021;10(7):2614–8.
17. Jensen KO, Lempert M, Sprengel K, et al. Is there any difference in the outcome of geriatric and non-geriatric severely injured patients? - a seven-year, retrospective, observational cohort study with matched-pair analysis. J Clin Med. 2020;9(11):3544.
18. Schipa C, Luca E, Ripa M, et al. Preoperative evaluation of the elderly patient. Saudi J Anaesth. 2023;17(4):482–90.
19. Peden CJ, Aggarwal G, Aitken RJ, et al. Guidelines for perioperative care for emergency laparotomy Enhanced Recovery After Surgery (ERAS) Society recommendations: part 1 – preoperative: diagnosis, rapid assessment and optimization. World J Surg. 2021;45(5):1272–90.
20. Kennedy CA, Shipway D, Barry K. Frailty and emergency abdominal surgery: a systematic review and meta-analysis. Surgeon. 2022;20(6):e307–14.
21. Castillo-Angeles M, Cooper Z, Jarman MP, et al. Association of frailty with morbidity and mortality in emergency general surgery by procedural risk level. JAMA Surg. 2021;156(1):68–74.
22. Van Zundert TCRV, Gatt SP, van Zundert AAJ. Anesthesia and perioperative pain relief in the frail elderly patient. Saudi J Anaesth. 2023;17(4):566–74.
23. Alghamdi AS, Almuzayyen H, Chowdhury T. The elderly in the post-anesthesia care unit. Saudi J Anaesth. 2023;17(4):540–9.
24. Nordquist D, Halaszynski TM. Perioperative multimodal anesthesia using regional techniques in the aging surgical patient. Pain Res Treat. 2014;2014:902174.
25. Al Harbi MK, Alshaghroud SM, Aljahdali MM, et al. Regional anesthesia for geriatric population. Saudi J Anaesth. 2023;17(4):523–32.
26. Novak-Jankovič V. Regional anaesthesia for the elderly patients. Period Biol. 2013;115(2):119–23.
27. Greenberg B, Jiang S, Nadler A. Postoperative protocols for older adults undergoing emergency surgery: a scoping review. Can J Surg. 2024;67(2):E149–57.
28. Coccolini F, Corradi F, Sartelli M, et al. Postoperative pain management in non-traumatic emergency general surgery: WSES-GAIS-SIAARTI-AAST guidelines. World J Emerg Surg. 2022;17(1):50.
29. van Dijk JF, Zaslansky R, van Boekel RLM, et al. Postoperative pain and age: a retrospective cohort association study. Anesthesiology. 2021;135(6):1104–19.
30. Vilches-Moraga A, Fox J. Geriatricians and the older emergency general surgical patient: proactive assessment and patient centred interventions. Salford-POP-GS Aging Clin Exp Res. 2018;30(3):277–82.

31. Assolari F, Mancin S, Lopane D, et al. Advanced practice nursing in surgery: a scoping review of roles, responsibilities, and educational programs. Int Nurs Rev. 2025;72(3):e13045.
32. Partridge JSL, Ryan J, Dhesi JK, et al. New guidelines for the perioperative care of people living with frailty undergoing elective and emergency surgery - a commentary. Age Ageing. 2022;51(11):afac237.
33. Esquiroz Lizaur I, Zambom-Ferraresi F, Zambom-Ferraresi F, et al. Postoperative physical rehabilitation in the elderly patient after emergency surgery. Influence on functional, cognitive and quality of live recovery: study protocol for a randomized clinical trial. Trials. 2024;25(1):584.
34. Soleman J, Ullmann M, Greuter L, et al. Mortality and outcome in elderly patients undergoing emergent or elective cranial surgery. World Neurosurg. 2021;146:e575–89.
35. Parmar KL, Law J, Carter B, et al. Frailty in older patients undergoing emergency laparotomy: results from the UK observational emergency laparotomy and frailty (ELF) study. Ann Surg. 2021;273(4):709–18.
36. Gottesman D, McIsaac DI. Frailty and emergency surgery: identification and evidence-based care for vulnerable older adults. Anaesthesia. 2022;77(12):1430–8.
37. Patrizio E, Zambon A, Mazzola P, et al. Assessing the mortality risk in older patients hospitalized with a diagnosis of sepsis: the role of frailty and acute organ dysfunction. Aging Clin Exp Res. 2022;34(10):2335–43.

Robotic Surgery

13

Carlo Alberto Schena, Francesco Marchegiani, Paolo Carcoforo, and Nicola de'Angelis

13.1 Introduction

Robotic surgery has emerged over the past three decades as one of the most significant technological innovations in operative medicine. The first clinical procedures were performed in the mid-1990s using early prototypes. The da Vinci Surgical System® (Intuitive Surgical, Sunnyvale, CA, USA) received FDA approval in 2000 for general laparoscopic surgery. Its adoption accelerated rapidly in the 2000s, first in urology, particularly radical prostatectomy, and subsequently spreading into gynecology, general surgery, and thoracic surgery. By 2023, more than ten million robotic operations had been performed, with over 7700 systems installed across more than 70 countries [1–3]. The rationale behind robotic surgery is to overcome the intrinsic limitations of conventional laparoscopy, such as two-dimensional vision, rigid instruments, tremor amplification, by offering stable three-dimensional magnified vision, articulated wristed instruments with seven degrees of freedom, tremor filtration, and motion scaling, together with an ergonomic surgeon console.

C. A. Schena
Department of Surgery, Fondazione Poliambulanza, Brescia, Italy

Department of Translational Medicine and LTTA Centre, University of Ferrara, Ferrara, Italy

F. Marchegiani
Unit of Colorectal and Digestive Surgery, DIGEST Department, Beaujon University Hospital (AP-HP), University Paris Cité, Paris, France
e-mail: francesco.marchegiani@aphp.fr

P. Carcoforo
Breast Surgery Unit, Ferrara University Hospital, Cona, Ferrara, Italy
e-mail: ccf@unife.it

N. de'Angelis (✉)
Unit of General, Oncologic, and Robotic Minimally-Invasive Surgery, Department of Surgery, Fondazione Poliambulanza, Brescia, Italy
e-mail: nic.deangelis@yahoo.it

P. Carcoforo, F. Catena (eds.), *Geriatric Surgery*, Updates in Surgery,
https://doi.org/10.1007/978-3-032-24281-5_13

These features are particularly advantageous in confined anatomical regions, such as the pelvis or mediastinum, and in complex reconstructive steps that require precise suturing.

Initially dominated by the da Vinci® system, the field is now entering a new phase of competition and diversification. Marchegiani et al. recently reviewed emerging robotic platforms and highlighted the Versius® (CMR Surgical, UK), Senhance® (Asensus, USA/Italy), Hinotori® (Medicaroid, Japan), Revo-i® (Meere Company, Korea), and the Single-Port da Vinci SP® as alternatives increasingly gaining approval and clinical use [4]. These systems aim to reduce costs, improve ergonomics, and broaden the accessibility of robotic assistance.

Robotic surgery's expansion has had a profound impact across specialties [5–12]:

- Urology remains the strongest field, with robotic-assisted radical prostatectomy now the standard of care in many countries, and applications extending to nephrectomy and cystectomy.
- Gynecology has widely adopted robotic hysterectomy and myomectomy, especially for complex or oncologic cases.
- Thoracic surgery increasingly employs robotic lobectomy and mediastinal resections.
- General and colorectal surgery represent rapidly expanding domains, with robotic colectomy, proctectomy, gastrectomy, and hernia repair demonstrating feasibility and growing adoption.

For the elderly, these technical advantages may be particularly relevant, as minimizing operative trauma and reducing conversions can lead to lower complication rates, faster recovery, and potentially preserved independence.

13.1.1 The Geriatric Surgical Patient

Older adults are heterogeneous. Frailty, cognitive status, nutrition, sarcopenia, comorbidity burden, and social support are stronger predictors of surgical outcomes than chronological age. The Italian multi-society consensus for elderly rectal cancer care recommends systematic geriatric assessment, prehabilitation, and tailored pathways, highlighting that fit older adults can achieve oncologic outcomes comparable to younger counterparts, while vulnerable or frail patients require individualized goals and strategies [13]. The multicenter GOSAFE cohort, comprising 977 patients aged 70 years and older, demonstrated the feasibility and clinical value of tracking functional trajectories and patient-reported outcomes following cancer surgery in older adults, thereby reframing the need for encompassing independence and quality of life as main endpoints in this cohort of patients [14].

13.2 Safety, Feasibility, and Effectiveness of Robotic Surgery in the Elderly

13.2.1 Overall Safety Across Specialties

Age itself does not contraindicate robotic surgery when selection and optimization are appropriate. A summary of the main studies on robotic surgery in elderly patients is presented in Table 13.1.

Table 13.1 Main studies on robotic surgery in elderly patients

Author (Year)	Population (Age cut-off)	Specialty	Study type	Main findings
Xue et al. [15] BMC Geriatr	111 (≥80 year)	Colorectal	R	Robotic lower blood loss, similar conversion, morbidity and 3y OS/DFS
Hannan et al. [16] Int J Med Robot	162 (<65, ≥65 year)	Colorectal	R	No differences in complications, anastomotic leaks, mortality
Thompson et al. [17] J Robot Surg	179 (≥80 year)	Colorectal	R	Shorter hospital stay, lower conversion, similar complications and oncologic adequacy with robotics
de'Angelis et al. [18] J Laparoendosc Adv Surg Tech	86 (≥70 year)	Colorectal	R + PSM	Robotic has longer operative times but no differences in morbidity and oncological outcomes
Topal et al. [19] Tech Coloproctol	134 (<79, ≥70 year)	Colorectal	R	Comparable operative time, staging, LN yield and pathology; elderly had higher stoma rates
Van Eetvelde et al. [20] J Geriatr Oncol	231 (<70, 70–79, 80–89, ≥90 year)	Colorectal	R	No differences in major morbidity or cancer-specific survival across ages. OS declined with age
Fortuna et al. [21] Cancers	143 (<75, ≥75 year)	Gastric	R	Similar severe complications, reoperation, mortality, LN yield, LOS
Yüksel et al. [22] Eur Rev Med Pharmacol Sci	68 (<79, ≥70 year)	Gastric	R	Equivalent operative time, morbidity, LN harvest, LOS
Marshall et al. (2024) [23] Surg Endosc	628 (<65, ≥65 year)	Gastric	R	Elderly had similar outcomes and comparable symptom control
Mederos et al. (2022) [24] HPB (Oxford)	2502, 725 after PSM (≥75 year)	Pancreatic	R + PSM	Similar complications, shorter LOS, higher readmission in robotic vs. open PD
Collins et al. (2023) [25] Ann Surg	2128, 1109 after PSM (≥65 year)	Abdominal wall	R + PSM	Robotic vs. open VHR: Shorter LOS, equivalent complications, better QoL at 1 year

DFS disease-free survival, *LN* lymph nodes, *LOS* length of stay, *OS* overall survival, *PD* pancreaticoduodenectomy, *PSM* propensity score matching, *QoL* quality of life, *R* retrospective, *VHR* ventral hernia repair

13.2.1.1 Colorectal Surgery

Evidence in colorectal cancer (CRC) is among the most mature. Xue et al. analyzed 111 octogenarians with CRC and found that robotic surgery halved intraoperative blood loss compared with laparoscopy (mean 76.9 mL vs. 161.6 mL, $p = 0.025$) with no differences in conversion, postoperative morbidity, or 3-year disease-free and overall survival [15]. In a single-center experience, Hannan et al. compared 89 elderly (aged ≥65 years) vs. 73 non-elderly patients undergoing robotic colorectal resections and observed no significant differences in postoperative complications, leaks, reoperations, or mortality. The median length of stay was longer in the elderly (median 7 vs. 6 days, $p = 0.007$). Octogenarian outcomes compared favorably with younger patients [16]. From a high-volume cancer center, Thompson et al. evaluated 179 patients aged ≥80 years undergoing minimally invasive colectomy and reported shorter length of stay (median 5 vs. 6 days, $p < 0.001$) and lower conversion rates (3% vs. 17%, $p = 0.002$) with a robotic approach compared with laparoscopy, with no compromise in complications or oncologic endpoints [17]. A contemporary review concluded that robotic colorectal surgery in older adults is safe and feasible, often with lower conversion, earlier bowel recovery, and shorter hospitalization, while oncologic quality is maintained despite generally longer operative times [26]. de'Angelis et al. conducted a propensity score-matched analysis on 86 patients aged ≥70 years undergoing colorectal cancer resection, comparing laparoscopic and robotic approaches. They reported that robotic procedures were associated with longer operative times (300 vs. 215 min, $p = 0.03$), but no significant differences in postoperative complications, conversion rates, blood loss, length of stay, or 90-day mortality. Oncological radicality was comparable, with more than 95% R0 resections, and similar overall and disease-free survival at 1, 2, and 3 years between groups. The authors concluded that robotic colorectal surgery in elderly patients is safe and oncologically equivalent to laparoscopy, despite longer operative times [18]. Topal et al. compared outcomes in ≥70-year-old rectal cancer patients versus younger counterparts. The study found comparable operative time, tumor staging, lymph-node yield, and pathological outcomes, though elderly patients had a higher stoma rate, supporting the safety and feasibility of robotic surgery in this group [19]. A comprehensive systematic review and meta-analysis by Gahunia et al., including 48 studies and over 34,000 patients (with 722 elderly robotic cases), found that robotic surgery in high-risk and elderly populations is associated with longer operative times but significantly lower conversion rates and shorter hospital stays compared to laparoscopy [27]. Finally, a recent age-stratified cohort of robot-assisted colon resections, including patients aged <70, 70–79, 80–89, and ≥ 90 years, reported no differences in 30-day major morbidity or 90-day mortality across age groups. Overall morbidity ($p = 0.02$), length of hospital stay ($p < 0.001$), and days to full mobility ($p = 0.003$) were increased in patients aged 70 years and older for right-sided colon surgery, whereas definitive stoma ($p = 0.03$), length of stay ($p = 0.008$), days to soft diet ($p = 0.07$) and to full mobility ($p = 0.045$) were increased for left-sided colon surgery. Cancer-specific survival did not differ by age, whereas 3-year and 5-year overall survival declined with age ($p < 0.001$), reflecting competing non-cancer mortality [20].

13.2.1.2 Upper Gastrointestinal Surgery

In gastric cancer, Fortuna et al. examined 143 robotic gastrectomies and showed that patients ≥75 years had similar rates of severe complications (Clavien–Dindo ≥III), reoperation, 30-day mortality, lymph-node yield, and median length of stay compared with younger patients, supporting feasibility without oncologic compromise [21]. In another institutional cohort comparing patients aged ≥70 years vs. <70 years, robotic gastrectomy produced similar operative times, complication rates, 90-day readmissions, lymph nodes harvested, and hospital stay. A single 30-day mortality occurred in the elderly group [22]. Beyond oncologic gastrectomy, a large cohort (2009–2023) of robotic anti-reflux surgery showed that among 190 elderly (≥65 years) of 628 patients, complications were no worse than in younger adults, with similar symptom relief and no increases in readmission or reoperation rate. Operative time was longer in the geriatric group (132 vs. 104.5 min, $p < 0.001$) [23].

13.2.1.3 Hepato-Pancreato-Biliary Surgery

Pancreaticoduodenectomy (PD) remains a high-risk operation in any age group. Using the NSQIP (National Surgical Quality Improvement Program) database, Mederos et al. propensity-score matched patients aged ≥75 years undergoing robot-assisted and open PD. The authors found broadly similar complication profiles, shorter length of stay (median 8 [interquartile range, IQR 6–11] vs. 8 [IQR 7–13] days, $p = 0.003$), but higher readmissions (28.1% vs. 17.7%, $p = 0.02$) for robotic cases, concluding that robotic PD appears safe in carefully selected elderly patients while highlighting the need for prospective studies [24].

13.2.1.4 Abdominal Wall Surgery

Using a national hernia registry and propensity matching, Collins et al. compared robotic versus open retromuscular ventral hernia repair in older adults (≥65 years). Robotic repair yielded a much shorter hospital stay (median 1 vs. 4 days, $p < 0.01$) with equivalent 30-day complications and readmissions. Notably, 1-year quality of life was modestly higher after robotics, supporting it as a valid option in selected elderly [25].

13.2.2 Comparative Effectiveness in Older Adults

Comparative data consistently demonstrate that robotic approaches are not inferior to laparoscopy or open surgery in elderly patients. In CRC, robotic surgery in patients aged 65–80 years and older maintains oncologic adequacy while reducing conversion and blood loss, with a length of stay equal to or shorter than that of laparoscopic comparators in several series [15–17, 26]. In gastric surgery, robotic gastrectomy yields equivalent severe complication rates and lymph-node yields in patients aged 70–75 years and older compared to younger cohorts, supporting its oncologic validity [21, 22] In hepato-pancreato-biliary surgery (HPB), robotic PD in patients ≥75 years yields shorter hospitalization times compared to open surgery, at the cost of more readmissions, with overall complication profiles similar in propensity-matched analyses [24]. In abdominal wall surgery, robotic repair offers significantly shorter hospitalization and equivalent safety compared to open approaches [25]. Functionally, the GOSAFE study underlines that independence and recovery of baseline function are critical outcomes in the elderly [14]. By enabling minimally invasive access with lower conversion rates, robotics plausibly supports these goals, although dedicated randomized geriatric trials are still needed. Another practical advantage of robotic platforms is the capacity to maintain exposure at lower insufflation pressures (i.e., "low-impact pneumoperitoneum"), which can reduce cardiopulmonary load. A recent anesthesiology review recommends using the lowest feasible pneumoperitoneum pressure and minimizing extreme positioning in the elderly [28]. Clinically, the lower conversion rates seen with robotic colectomy in octogenarians, together with reduced blood loss, likely mitigate the systemic inflammatory insult of unplanned laparotomy and may help explain the consistent signals of shorter stays without excess morbidity [17].

13.2.3 Cost-Effectiveness and Health-System Perspectives

The economics of robotic surgery remain one of the most debated topics. Peng et al.'s bibliometric analysis highlighted that the health economics of robotic surgery is a rapidly expanding field, but research remains unbalanced, with the majority of publications originating from the USA and Europe and few cost-utility studies dedicated to the elderly [3]. Multiple analyses show that robotic procedures are consistently more expensive than laparoscopic ones [29]. Added costs are attributed to system amortization, maintenance contracts, and disposable instruments [30]. However, some studies argue that robotic surgery can achieve indirect cost savings in certain populations. Reduced conversion rates, fewer complications, and shorter length of stay may offset some of the higher procedural costs [31]. In addition, the value of robotics is maximized in high-volume centers with structured training programs, where efficiency gains and complication reduction can substantially improve cost-effectiveness. Since elderly patients are more prone to complications and prolonged hospitalizations, they might represent the subgroup where robotics offers the greatest relative value. A very recent systematic review and meta-analysis of randomized controlled trials (RCTs), specifically focused on older adults aged ≥60 years, has provided important evidence. The authors synthesized five RCTs involving 666 patients and showed that robotic surgery incurred higher total costs compared with open or laparoscopic procedures (mean difference [MD] \$ 1316; 95% CI: 10.68–2622.08, $p = 0.048$, $I^2 = 92.5\%$), mainly driven by operating room expenses. However, hospitalization costs were slightly lower (but not statistically significant), and quality-adjusted life year (QALY) gains were significantly higher in robotic groups (MD 0.01; 95% CI: 0.00–0.02, $p = 0.01$, $I^2 = 0\%$) [32]. Further analyses indicated that robotic surgery achieved an incremental cost-effectiveness ratio between \$ 14,925 and \$ 28,860 per QALY, values well below the commonly accepted threshold of \$ 50,000 [32]. These findings suggest that although robotic surgery has higher upfront costs, it can be economically justified in older adults when long-term outcomes and functional recovery are taken into account. This is consistent with the hypothesis that the elderly, being more vulnerable to complications, prolonged stays, and loss of independence, may represent a population where robotic surgery yields the highest relative value. At the system level, health economic sustainability depends strongly on case volume and institutional efficiency. High-volume centers can dilute fixed costs and achieve greater cost-effectiveness.

In conclusion, while costs remain a challenge, emerging geriatric-focused analyses suggest that robotic surgery can be cost-effective in older patients by improving quality of life and functional recovery, and by reducing long-term healthcare utilization.

13.3 Future Directions in Geriatric Robotic Surgery

The next decade will bring greater competition among robotic platforms, likely reducing costs and broadening access. Integration of artificial intelligence, augmented reality, fluorescence-guided surgery, and tele-surgery is expected to enhance safety and precision. Importantly, clinical trials should incorporate elderly and frail patients to provide robust data on functional and quality-of-life outcomes.

13.4 Conclusions

Robotic surgery is safe and feasible in elderly and very elderly patients when selection is guided by frailty and comorbidity rather than age alone. Across colorectal, gastric, urologic, abdominal wall, and selected HPB procedures, robotics reduces conversions and blood loss, shortens hospitalization, and preserves oncologic adequacy. The ability to operate with low-impact pneumoperitoneum is particularly relevant to geriatric physiology. While costs and access remain significant barriers, robotic surgery has the potential to mitigate surgical stress and improve recovery in older adults. Future studies must address cost-utility in elderly populations and prioritize patient-centered endpoints such as function and independence.

References

1. Sheetz KH, Claflin J, Dimick JB. Trends in the adoption of robotic surgery for common surgical procedures. JAMA Netw Open. 2020;3(1):e1918911.
2. Diana M, Marescaux J. Robotic surgery. Br J Surg. 2015;102(2):e15–28.
3. Peng Y, Liu Y, Lai S, et al. Global trends and prospects in health economics of robotic surgery: a bibliometric analysis. Int J Surg. 2023;109(12):3896–904.
4. Marchegiani F, Siragusa L, Zadoroznyj A, et al. New robotic platforms in general surgery: what's the current clinical scenario? Medicina (Kaunas). 2023;59(7):1264.
5. Brassetti A, Ragusa A, Tedesco F, et al. Robotic surgery in urology: history from PROBOT® to HUGO™. Sensors (Basel). 2023;23(16):7104.

6. Han ES, Advincula AP. Robotic surgery: advancements and inflection points in the field of gynecology. Obstet Gynecol Clin N Am. 2021;48(4):759–76.
7. Schwartz G, Sancheti M, Blasberg J. Robotic thoracic surgery. Surg Clin North Am. 2020;100(2):237–48.
8. Bianchi G, Gavriilidis P, Martínez-Pérez A, et al. Robotic multiquadrant colorectal procedures: a single-center experience and a systematic review of the literature. Front Surg. 2022;9:991704.
9. de'Angelis N, Schena CA, Azzolina D, et al. Histopathological outcomes of transanal, robotic, open, and laparoscopic surgery for rectal cancer resection. A Bayesian network meta-analysis of randomized controlled trials. Eur J Surg Oncol. 2025;51(1):109481.
10. de'Angelis N, Schena CA, Moszkowicz D, et al. Robotic surgery for inguinal and ventral hernia repair: a systematic review and meta-analysis. Surg Endosc. 2024;38(1):24–46.
11. de'Angelis N, Marchegiani F, Martínez-Pérez A, et al. Robotic, transanal, and laparoscopic total mesorectal excision for locally advanced mid/low rectal cancer: European multicentre, propensity score-matched study. BJS Open. 2024;8(3):zrae044.
12. de'Angelis N, Schena CA, Espin-Basany E, et al. Robotic versus laparoscopic right colectomy for nonmetastatic pT4 colon cancer: a European multicentre propensity score-matched analysis. Color Dis. 2024;26(8):1569–83.
13. Podda M, Sylla P, Baiocchi G, et al. Multidisciplinary management of elderly patients with rectal cancer: recommendations from the SICG (Italian Society of Geriatric Surgery), SIFIPAC (Italian Society of Surgical Pathophysiology), SICE (Italian Society of Endoscopic Surgery and new technologies), and the WSES (World Society of Emergency Surgery) International Consensus Project. World J Emerg Surg. 2021;16(1):35.
14. Montroni I, Rostoft S, Spinelli A, et al. GOSAFE – Geriatric Oncology Surgical Assessment and Functional rEcovery after surgery: early analysis on 977 patients. J Geriatr Oncol. 2020;11(2):244–55.
15. Xue Y, Li S, Guo S, et al. Evaluation of the advantages of robotic versus laparoscopic surgery in elderly patients with colorectal cancer. BMC Geriatr. 2023;23(1):105.
16. Hannan E, Feeney G, Fahad Ullah M, et al. Robotic colorectal surgery in elderly patients: a single-centre experience. Int J Med Robot. 2022;18(5):e2431.
17. Thompson HM, Williams H, Omer DM, et al. Comparison of short-term outcomes and survival between minimally invasive colectomy and open colectomy in patients 80 years of age and older. J Robot Surg. 2023;17(4):1857–65.
18. de'Angelis N, Abdalla S, Bianchi G, et al. Robotic versus laparoscopic colorectal cancer surgery in elderly patients: a propensity score match analysis. J Laparoendosc Adv Surg Tech A. 2018;28(11):1334–45.
19. Topal U, Yüksel S, Songür MZ, et al. Safety and feasibility of robotic surgery in geriatric patients with rectal cancer. Tech Coloproctol. 2024;28(1):152.
20. Van Eetvelde E, Verweirder M, Decoster L, Jacobs-Tulleneers-Thevissen D. Outcome of robotic colon surgery in older patients with colon cancer. J Geriatr Oncol. 2025;16(3):102205.
21. Fortuna L, Staderini F, Coratti F, Cianchi F. Comparison of short-term outcomes after robotic surgery for gastric cancer in elderly and younger patients: a retrospective cohort study. Cancers (Basel). 2024;16(16):2849.
22. Yüksel S, Topal U, Songur MZ, et al. Robotic gastrectomy is safe in geriatric patients with gastric cancer: a retrospective cohort study. Eur Rev Med Pharmacol Sci. 2024;28(8):3041–7.
23. Marshall TE, Alqamish M, Salehi N, et al. Safety and efficacy of robotic anti-reflux surgery in geriatric patients: a comparative analysis. Surg Endosc. 2024;38(9):5285–91.
24. Mederos MA, Starr S, Park JY, et al. Robotic versus open pancreaticoduodenectomy in elderly patients: a propensity score-matched analysis. HPB (Oxford). 2023;25(3):301–10.
25. Collins CE, Renshaw S, Huang LC, Phillips S, Gure TR, Poulose B. Robotic vs. open approach for older adults undergoing retromuscular ventral hernia repair. Ann Surg. 2023;277(4):697–703.
26. Teo NZ, Ngu JCY. Robotic surgery in elderly patients with colorectal cancer: review of the current literature. World J Gastrointest Surg. 2023;15(6):1040–7.

27. Gahunia S, Wyatt J, Powell SG, et al. Robotic-assisted versus laparoscopic surgery for colorectal cancer in high-risk patients: a systematic review and meta-analysis. Tech Coloproctol. 2025;29(1):98.
28. Aceto P, Galletta C, Cambise C, et al. Challenges for anaesthesia for robotic-assisted surgery in the elderly: a narrative review. Eur J Anaesthesiol Intensive Care. 2023;2(2):e0019.
29. Childers CP, Maggard-Gibbons M. Estimation of the acquisition and operating costs for robotic surgery. JAMA. 2018;320(8):835–6.
30. Higgins RM, Frelich MJ, Bosler ME, Gould JC. Cost analysis of robotic versus laparoscopic general surgery procedures. Surg Endosc. 2017;31(1):185–92.
31. Ielpo B, Podda M, Burdio F, et al. Cost-effectiveness of robotic vs. laparoscopic surgery for different surgical procedures: protocol for a prospective, multicentric study (ROBOCOSTES). Front Surg. 2022;9:866041.
32. Tang Y, Dou B. Cost-effectiveness analysis of robotic surgery in healthcare for older individuals: a systematic review based on randomized controlled trials. Front Public Health. 2025;13:1614654.

Day Surgery, One Day Surgery

14

Piergaspare Palumbo, Bruno Perotti, Riccardo Centamore, and Antonio Biondi

14.1 Introduction

Eurostat shows that Italy is the oldest country in the EU, with a median population age of 48.7 years on 1 January 2024 (EU average 44.7 years). It has the fastest aging rate in Europe, with an increase of 4 years per decade, and the highest old-age dependency ratio (65+ compared to those aged 15–64), with over a third of the population over 65 [1].

The spread of day surgery units is a progressively growing phenomenon throughout Italy and Europe and can rightfully be considered one of the major revolutions in surgery over the last 20 years. Demand for day surgery services has also been steadily growing among the elderly population, who are eager to return home early. However, some resistance, at least initially, has been expressed by caregivers, who have expressed concerns about having to take on the responsibility of caring for the elderly patient in the postoperative period.

In general, the objectives of day surgery include:

- Improving clinical and organizational appropriateness, reducing inappropriate and prolonged hospitalizations and facilitating early recovery and a rapid return to normal lifestyle, thus reducing psychological stress.

P. Palumbo (✉)
Department of Surgery, Sapienza University of Rome, Rome, Italy
e-mail: piergaspare.palumbo@uniroma1.it

B. Perotti
General Surgery Unit, Versilia Hospital – AUSL Toscana Nord-Ovest, Lido di Camaiore, LU, Italy
e-mail: bruno.perotti86@gmail.com

R. Centamore · A. Biondi
Department of General Surgery and Medical Surgical Specialties, University of Catania, Catania, Italy
e-mail: centamore.riccardo@gmail.com; abiondi@unict.it

P. Carcoforo, F. Catena (eds.), *Geriatric Surgery*, Updates in Surgery,
https://doi.org/10.1007/978-3-032-24281-5_14

- Reducing the incidence of nosocomial infections.
- Facilitating the elimination of waiting lists and the optimization of available resources.

Therefore, day surgery arises from the need to combine safety, quality, and cost-effectiveness.

Elderly patients are often frail, and a shorter treatment time can be beneficial. Naturally, they must be managed through an appropriate organizational and management system, and surgical treatment must be personalized.

For this reason, day surgery is a setting that requires rigorous and highly efficient organization.

Specifically, the system's governance must consider all phases of the care pathway, from planning to the implementation of procedures, both preoperatively and postoperatively, as well as the evaluation of results.

Day surgery refers to "the possibility of performing, with appropriate clinical, organizational, and administrative methods, surgical interventions or even invasive and semi-invasive diagnostic and/or therapeutic procedures in a hospital setting limited to daytime hours only, under local, loco-regional, or general anesthesia. To meet the specific care needs of hospitalizations requiring an overnight stay, regions may, according to their own needs and organizational methods, avail themselves of either ordinary one-day hospitalization or day surgery followed by an overnight stay".

Knowledge of regulatory frameworks is essential. In Italy, the main references are the Agreement between the State, the Regions, and the Autonomous Provinces of August 1, 2002 (Accordo Stato—Regioni—Province Autonome), and Ministerial Decree No. 70 of April 2, 2017 (Decreto Ministeriale No. 70).

Furthermore, all Regions and Autonomous Provinces have issued specific regulations on the matter.

From a logistical standpoint, it is advisable for day surgery units to be separated from other care modalities, particularly long-stay hospitalization. Ease of access and management of the care process is closely linked to the separation of care flows, which should not overlap with other care pathways, which could lead to inappropriate interference in clinical and care pathways.

14.2 Day Surgery—How It Works

14.2.1 Pre-admission

Patient selection and admission are the initial and most delicate phase of a day surgery pathway.

The criteria taken into consideration must be made explicit, shared by the organization, and documented. The indication for surgery or procedure as a day surgery must consider clinical and social criteria.

14.2.1.1 Clinical Criteria

Among the clinical criteria, advanced age is not an absolute contraindication to day surgery procedures and even a person over 80 years of age can be admitted to day surgery. However, the patient's health status is of great importance, and the concept of clinical frailty must guide through the decision whether or not to include the patient in the process.

Surgery, even minor surgery, is in any case a trauma to the body, especially for the elderly, and it can lead to an imbalance in the patient's health, especially in the case of frail and elderly patients whose balance is already fragile and difficult to recover when lost.

In all cases, physiological mechanisms are triggered to compensate for the stress caused by the surgery, the so-called surgical stress response. The resources used to adapt to this condition must utilize all available physiological reserves, which may be insufficient for the adaptation process, precisely because of a frail condition. Therefore, maximum attention must be focused on the presence of comorbidities.

14.2.1.2 Risk Stratification

Postoperative complications in older adults represent a significant cause of increased hospital length of stay and patient distress despite major advances in surgical and anesthetic techniques and perioperative care. In addition, they can determine increased management costs.

Risk assessment in day surgery should resolve the following questions: does the rate of risk change when performing an operation on an outpatient rather than an inpatient basis, and what predictors of complications exist when surgery is performed on an outpatient basis [2]. Possible categories of complications include cardiac (cardiac arrest, myocardial infarction), respiratory (pneumonia, pulmonary embolism), renal insufficiency, neurological (cerebral vascular accident, coma), postoperative infection (deep or superficial surgical site wound infection, urinary tract infection, sepsis), deep vein thrombosis, and re-operation.

Risk stratification is assessed using various scoring systems, such as the American Society of Anesthesiologists (ASA) Physical Status Classification System, the Acute Physiology and Chronic Health Evaluation (APACHE-II), the Physiologic and Severity Score for the Enumeration of Mortality and Morbidity (POSSUM), and the Goldman Cardiac Risk Index [3].

Elderly adults are very frequently affected by cardiorespiratory diseases, particularly chronic obstructive pulmonary disease (COPD). Several studies demonstrate that asthma and COPD are associated with increased perioperative risk [2, 4]. These patients must be prepared with targeted therapies (antibiotic therapy, bronchodilators, respiratory physiotherapy). A significant reduction in forced expiratory volume in 1 s (FEV1 < 0.70) is considered predictive of increased postoperative pulmonary complications and mortality, and it is a criterion for exclusion from day surgery. On the other hand, patients without respiratory involvement do not require preoperative spirometry or specific preparation. Smoking cessation is effective in all cases, but only if started 6–8 weeks before surgery.

Obstructive sleep apnea (OSA) is a common sleep disorder characterized by total or partial airway obstruction during sleep. It is an independent risk factor and is often underestimated: however, it can be associated with serious complications. OSA can be assessed as mild, moderate, or severe. In unclear cases, preoperative polysomnography can be critical and determine inclusion criteria in day surgery.

Cardiovascular risk factors are common in elderly patients. Coronary artery disease (CAD), congestive heart failure (CHF), and severe valvular heart disease (particularly aortic stenosis) are associated with the onset of adverse events [5]. Currently, advances in treatment techniques and thorough preoperative assessment have significantly reduced the risk of complications, but it is necessary to carefully investigate the stability of angina and evaluate other associated risk factors, such as diabetes and hypertension. Of course, optimizing drug therapy is essential. Following the publication of Goldman's now dated Multifactorial Index of Cardiac Risk in noncardiac surgical procedures, newer algorithms may help assess cardiac risk [6, 7].

Patients with uncontrolled diabetes with elevated glycated hemoglobin levels show a greater risk of major postoperative complications than patients with glucose intolerance or those without diabetes. Although anemia is a condition often found in the elderly it needs to be identified and corrected before surgery. The anemic state in the preoperative period is closely associated with increased morbidity and postoperative mortality, so it can be considered a predictive factor.

Anticoagulant/antiplatelet therapy must be carefully evaluated. Discontinuation of aspirin is not required in day surgery procedures. However, discontinuation of NOACs (new oral anticoagulants) should be carefully considered, and, in some cases, replacement with low molecular weight heparin.

The ASA score is commonly considered a criterion for inclusion in day surgery procedures and for risk assessment. Patients classified as ASA I and II are generally eligible, and, after careful evaluation, even some ASA III patients, if the associated comorbidity appears to be stabilized. However, the ASA factor does not appear to be associated with unanticipated readmission after surgery, while nausea, vomiting, and pain are more significant [8]. In fact, some authors exclude ASA assessment from the inclusion criteria for day surgery procedures [9].

An important issue to consider when dealing with hospitalized elderly patients is stress management. Elderly patients, even those who are completely independent at home, experience distress once in the hospital following the onset of stress. In this state of distress, geriatric patients may exhibit two behaviors that fall within the "general adjustment syndrome", with depressive or, conversely, aggressive reactions. Prolonged hospitalization is sometimes accompanied by the onset of postoperative delirium, which causes serious distress for the patient, their family, and all healthcare workers.

In this sense, reducing hospital stay can minimize the risks of delirium and adjustment syndrome.

The preoperative anesthesiological evaluation must confirm the patient's eligibility for day surgery. The type of anesthesia must be identified and agreed upon, considering the elderly patient's frailty. Local or locoregional anesthesia should be preferred, as should ultrasound-guided peripheral blocks. Anticoagulation can sometimes hinder the implementation of this type of anesthesia. A laryngeal mask airway, where necessary, may be preferable to orotracheal intubation in cases of COPD or asthma. The type of anesthesia in cardiovascular conditions generally should minimize factors that increase oxygen consumption (hypertension, pain). Patients with a foreseeable need for prolonged hospitalization, even for observation or for drainage monitoring that cannot be managed at home, should be excluded.

Preoperative counseling, including that provided by nurses, is highly effective in reducing anxiety and anxiety related to hospitalization and the surgery, and it significantly increases patient satisfaction. Counseling can be easily performed via teleconsultation, and it is beneficial for elderly patients who can receive useful information directly at their home [10].

14.2.1.3 Social Criteria

In day surgery assessment, the patient is discharged to continue the recovery process at home, but certain requirements must be met to ensure discharge.

The caregiver is a key figure in the treatment process. They must be clearly identified and able to understand and follow the instructions given by healthcare professionals. From the preoperative stage, they must help the patient follow the instructions given, including which medications to take or stop, hygiene rules, and punctuality in keeping appointments. Correctly identifying the caregiver and their agreement to care for the patient is a prerequisite for admission to day surgery. The caregiver must be physically identified by the surgical facility staff. Sometimes, the elderly patient designates a relative (wife or husband) as the caregiver, who is also elderly and unable to care for the patient.

The patient must be reachable at all times, either by telephone, telemedicine, or in person by the doctor or nurse. Although complications at home are rare and, as mentioned, unplanned readmissions are unusual, the patient must be promptly reachable for a follow-up visit. The patient's home must therefore be within a reasonable distance from the surgical facility (maximum 1 h, preferably 30 min) and accessible without obstacles (difficult roads, snow) at all times. The patient's home must have hygiene standards compatible with the type of procedure performed.

14.2.2 Operative Day

The list of procedures permitted in day surgery is regulated by specific regulations. In Italy, the reference is the Prime Minister's Decree (DPCM) of January 12, 2017, followed and implemented through regional guidelines.

Informed consent is mandatory and must contain information regarding the type of procedure, the anesthesiological and surgical procedure, as well as information regarding the postoperative and home care plan. Detailed information is essential to achieve maximum patient compliance.

In conventional practice, preoperative fasting in its "*nihil per os*" (NPO) form from midnight the day before surgery is considered standard. This recommendation is strongly embedded in clinical practice and is justified in the attempt to prevent aspiration pneumonia. Several studies have refuted the claim that fasting provides an "empty stomach", confirming that during fasting the stomach can secrete up to 50 mL/h of gastric juice, and thus highlighting the limits of preoperative fasting and potential harmful effects.

Enhanced Recovery After Surgery (ERAS®) protocols have become widespread and implemented to reduce length of hospital stay by promoting early discharge, thereby limiting costs and increasing patient satisfaction. These protocols, now applied in many surgical procedures, originate from practices developed in day surgery. The cornerstones of the ERAS® protocol are preoperative counseling and education, opioid-sparing analgesia, nausea and vomiting prevention, fluid infusion reduction, pain control, early nutritional intake, and encouragement of early mobility. There is current evidence on the clinical importance of implementing an ERAS® protocol for ambulatory surgery [11].

Finally, it is essential that day surgery be "gentle", attentive to minimizing complications, and performed by experienced surgical teams.

14.2.3 Postoperative Phases

We can consider the immediate postoperative phase and the home care phase.

In the hours following surgery, the primary objectives are to restore the patient's independence and provide adequate pain control. Therefore, in addition to the necessary pharmacological therapies, it is important that the healthcare personnel, particularly nurses, help the patient regain deambulation and generally be attentive to the specific needs of the elderly patient, which may differ from those of younger patients. An excellent evaluation criterion during the course of treatment and upon discharge is the Post Anesthesia Discharge Scoring System [12] which takes into account six parameters:

1. Vital signs
2. Nausea, vomiting
3. Pain
4. Bleeding
5. Gait
6. Urination.

Each score is assigned a score from 0 (min) to 2 (max). The minimum score for a satisfactory return to independence is ≥9. However, for safety reasons, parameter 1 must always be equal to 2 and the other parameters ≥1. No parameter should be equal to 0.

Upon discharge, as mentioned, a comprehensive information brochure must be provided with the guidelines to follow and the main complications to be promptly communicated to the healthcare personnel.

Once discharged, the patient must be guaranteed continuity of care, particularly the availability of healthcare professionals. Availability must be provided by both doctors and nurses, according to the sequence established by the facility's regulations, and is generally achieved through telephone contact. In these instances, it is strongly recommended that a questionnaire be completed to serve as an objective recording system for patient-reported data. Telemedicine and image transmission can be of great help for remote patient assessment.

14.3 Conclusion

Day surgery is a process that can also be undertaken by elderly patients [13]. Risk identification is essential for perioperative risk reduction. Patients with comorbidities need careful preoperative evaluation by expert surgeons and anesthetists with day surgery experience and supported by an adequate healthcare facility [2]. The healthcare professionals' skill and an adequate surgical and anesthetic technique must be carefully considered, as well as the selection of patients to be admitted to day surgery units. A careful and experienced organization of the day surgery center can ensure the choice to treat elderly and frail patients as outpatients.

Day surgery for elderly patients has the advantage of enabling a choice of the most appropriate care setting for each individual, and encouraging clinical and organizational innovation, reducing waiting lists and combining quality, efficiency, and safety, and increasing patient satisfaction.

Naturally, eligibility criteria must be redefined as technology and risk management solutions advance. Not only clinical expertise, but also non-technical skills are crucial to optimally manage the patient journey. In this regard, new technologies and telemedicine can greatly assist in organizing and managing the care setting. Finally, careful attention is needed to evaluate outcomes and implement a continuous improvement program.

References

1. Eurostat. Demography of Europe – 2025 edition [Internet]. Eurostat; 2025 May [cited 2025 Dec 21]. Available from: https://ec.europa.eu/eurostat/web/products-interactive-publications/w/ks-01-24-025.
2. Bettelli G. High risk patients in day surgery. Minerva Anestesiol. 2009;75(5):259–68.
3. Ko FC. Preoperative frailty evaluation: a promising risk-stratification tool in older adults undergoing general surgery. Clin Ther. 2019;41(3):387–99.
4. Fortier J, Chung F, Su J. Unanticipated admission after ambulatory surgery – a prospective study. Can J Anaesth. 1998;45(7):612–9.
5. Handke J, Scholz AS, Dehne S, et al. Presepsin for pre-operative prediction of major adverse cardiovascular events in coronary heart disease patients undergoing noncardiac surgery: post hoc analysis of the Leukocytes and Cardiovascular Peri-operative Events-2 (LeukoCAPE-2) Study. Eur J Anaesthesiol. 2020;37(10):908–19.
6. Goldman L, Caldera DL, Nussbaum SR, et al. Multifactorial index of cardiac risk in noncardiac surgical procedures. N Engl J Med. 1977;297(16):845–50.

7. Caliskan B, Guldal G, Seker B, et al. Pre-operative cardiac risk assessment to predict mortality and intensive care admission in elderly patients scheduled for non-cardiac surgery: comparison of the revised cardiac and geriatric sensitive cardiac risk indices with cardiology-determined risk. Eur Arch Med Res. 2025;41(4):246–52.
8. Gold BS, Kitz DS, Lecky JH, Neuhaus JM. Unanticipated admission to the hospital following ambulatory surgery. JAMA. 1989;262(21):3008–10.
9. Gandhimani P, Jackson IJB. UK guidelines for day surgery. Surg Oxf. 2006;24(10):346–9.
10. Ozbek MN, Seyhan Ak E. The effect of preoperative tele-nursing counseling on anxiety and patient satisfaction in day surgery: a randomized controlled trial. J Perianesthesia Nurs. 2025;40(4):852–60.
11. Cukierman DS, Cata JP, Gan TJ. Enhanced recovery protocols for ambulatory surgery. Best Pract Res Clin Anaesthesiol. 2023;37(3):285–303.
12. Palumbo P, Tellan G, Perotti B, et al. Modified PADSS (Post Anaesthetic Discharge Scoring System) for monitoring outpatients discharge. Ann Ital Chir. 2013;84(6):661–5.
13. Palumbo P, Amatucci C, Perotti B, et al. Outpatient repair for inguinal hernia in elderly patients: still a challenge? Int J Surg. 2014;12(Suppl 2):S4–7.

Esophageal and Gastric Surgery for Cancer

15

Laura Fortuna, Francesco Coratti, Fabio Staderini, Federico Passagnoli, and Fabio Cianchi

15.1 Global Epidemiology and Demographics of Esophageal and Gastric Cancer

Esophageal cancer (EC) remains a major global health challenge, ranking as the seventh most common malignancy and the sixth leading cause of cancer-related mortality, with 511,000 new cases and 445,000 deaths reported in 2022 [1]. Its high mortality-to-incidence ratio reflects poor prognosis, particularly in locally advanced stages. Despite advances in diagnostics and therapy, the global five-year survival rate rarely exceeds 20% [2, 3].

Demographic shifts reveal an increasing proportion of elderly patients, with the median age at diagnosis approaching 68 years. Nearly one-third of cases occur in individuals ≥75 years, and 8% in those ≥85 [3, 4]. In countries with high life expectancy, such as Japan and the United States, the proportion of elderly patients undergoing esophagectomy has risen significantly—for instance, in Japan from 18% in 2011 to 25.4% in 2019 [5]. These trends highlight the need for treatment strategies specifically tailored to older populations.

Gastric cancer (GC) is the fifth most frequently diagnosed cancer and the fourth leading cause of cancer-related death worldwide. In 2020, 1.09 million new cases and 769,000 deaths were reported, corresponding to incidence and mortality rates of 11.1 and 7.7 per 100,000, respectively. Projections estimate 1.8 million cases and 1.3 million deaths annually by 2040.

GC incidence increases markedly after age 50, with peak rates between 65 and 85 years. Men are affected two to three times more often than women, likely due to environmental and hormonal factors. The highest burden is observed in East Asia—particularly China, Japan, and South Korea—which together account for

L. Fortuna (✉) · F. Coratti · F. Staderini · F. Passagnoli · F. Cianchi
Digestive Surgery Unit, Careggi University Hospital, Florence, Italy

Department of Experimental and Clinical Medicine, University of Florence, Florence, Italy
e-mail: laura9.fortuna@gmail.com; corattif@gmail.com; fabio.staderini@unifi.it; federico.passagnoli@unifi.it; fabio.cianchi@unifi.it

P. Carcoforo, F. Catena (eds.), *Geriatric Surgery*, Updates in Surgery,
https://doi.org/10.1007/978-3-032-24281-5_15

over 60% of global cases. In these regions, nationwide screening programs enable earlier detection and more effective interventions, whereas in Western countries, the absence of such programs results in a higher prevalence of advanced-stage diagnoses.

15.2 The Elderly Patient: Physiological and Clinical Considerations

Esophageal Surgery With aging comes a progressive decline in physiological reserve across multiple organ systems, a phenomenon that impacts tolerance to surgical and oncological therapies. Elderly patients frequently exhibit reduced cardiopulmonary capacity, impaired renal function, and diminished immune responsiveness—all of which compound the risks associated with esophagectomy, a procedure well recognized for its invasiveness and high postoperative morbidity.

Common clinical features among elderly EC patients include a higher prevalence of cardiovascular and pulmonary comorbidities, nutritional deficits, sarcopenia, and polypharmacy. These factors elevate perioperative risk and complicate recovery. In retrospective series, patients aged ≥75 years consistently demonstrate higher rates of cardiac events, postoperative delirium, and discharge to rehabilitation facilities, even when short-term outcomes such as anastomotic leakage and 30-day mortality are comparable to younger cohorts [6–9].

Despite these challenges, elderly patients may still achieve acceptable postoperative outcomes if appropriately selected based on functional and physiological assessments rather than age alone [10, 11]. Therefore, individualized evaluation remains essential to ensuring oncologic efficacy without undue harm.

Gastric Surgery With the global increase in life expectancy, the proportion of GC patients in older age groups has significantly risen. Multicenter data from South Korea revealed that individuals aged 71 and older constituted nearly 29% of all GC cases in 2019, up from 9% in 1995. The aging process is accompanied by a progressive decline in the physiological function of multiple organ systems. Cellular senescence, chronic inflammation, oxidative stress, and the accumulation of DNA damage contribute to impaired homeostasis and diminished capacity to withstand physiological stress.

More than 60% of elderly individuals live with multiple chronic conditions, including cardiovascular disease, diabetes, chronic respiratory diseases, and renal insufficiency. These comorbidities complicate perioperative management and amplify surgical risk. Elderly patients often present with atypical symptomatology and delayed diagnosis, increasing the likelihood of presenting with advanced disease.

15.3 Frailty: A Central Determinant in the Elderly with Esophageal and Gastric Cancer

Frailty, a multidimensional syndrome marked by reduced physiological reserves and increased vulnerability to stressors, is a critical determinant of surgical outcomes in elderly patients. Unlike chronological age, it more accurately predicts postoperative complications, delayed recovery, and mortality. The European Society for Clinical Nutrition and Metabolism (ESPEN) defines frailty as a state of heightened vulnerability due to cumulative physiological decline.

Assessment tools integrating nutrition, sarcopenia, cognition, and physical performance outperform conventional comorbidity indices (e.g., American Society of Anesthesiologists [ASA] score, Charlson Comorbidity Index) in predicting surgical risk. Instruments such as the G8 screening tool, Comprehensive Geriatric Assessment (CGA), Fried's Frailty Phenotype (FP), Clinical Frailty Scale (CFS), and Frailty Index (FI) have shown strong predictive validity in oncogeriatric populations. The reported prevalence of frailty in GC patients ranges from 10% to 71%, with a pooled estimate of ~29%.

Frailty consistently correlates with adverse outcomes, including higher rates of postoperative complications, prolonged hospitalization, readmission, long-term care dependency, and increased mortality (up to 3.3-fold higher than non-frail patients). It also negatively affects quality of life (QoL), particularly mobility, independence, and psychological well-being. Importantly, frailty is a modifiable risk factor: prehabilitation strategies – nutritional optimization, exercise, and management of comorbidities – may enhance resilience and improve postoperative results.

15.3.1 Risk Factors and Predictors of Preoperative Frailty

Esophageal Surgery Several clinical and biological parameters are associated with an increased risk of frailty in elderly EC patients. These include:

- Age ≥75 years: although not synonymous with frailty, advanced age correlates with a higher probability of functional decline.
- Low body mass index (BMI) or sarcopenia: frequently observed in EC patients due to dysphagia-induced malnutrition.
- Poor Eastern Cooperative Oncology Group (ECOG) or WHO performance status (≥2).
- Hypoalbuminemia and low prealbumin levels, reflecting nutritional and inflammatory status.
- Pre-existing comorbidities, particularly congestive heart failure, chronic obstructive pulmonary disease, and chronic kidney disease.
- Cognitive impairment or history of falls, which may signal underlying frailty and predict postoperative delirium.

Recognition and quantification of these risk factors can guide clinical decision-making and inform the risk-benefit assessment for aggressive treatment modalities.

Gastric Surgery A comprehensive meta-analysis has identified several independent predictors of preoperative frailty in elderly gastric cancer patients:

- Demographic factors: chronological age, active smoking, and educational attainment were significantly associated with frailty. Notably, individuals with a high school education or higher exhibited lower frailty risk, potentially due to better health literacy, cognitive reserve, and lifestyle factors.
- Physiological and biochemical indicators: hypoalbuminemia and anemia are strongly associated with frailty. Serum albumin reflects nutritional and inflammatory status, while hemoglobin levels are critical for oxygen delivery and muscle function. Albumin levels below 3.5 g/dL and hemoglobin concentrations under 12 g/dL are frequently observed in frail individuals.
- Disease-specific variables: advanced tumor stage (III–IV), a Charlson Comorbidity Index (CCI) score ≥3, ECOG performance status >2, and an ASA score >2 are potent predictors of frailty. Nutritional risk, as assessed by validated tools such as the Mini Nutritional Assessment (MNA), and sleep disturbances also contribute significantly.

These findings emphasize the multifactorial nature of frailty and underscore the necessity for a multidisciplinary preoperative assessment that includes nutritional, physical, cognitive, and psychosocial domains.

15.4 Surgical Management in the Elderly: Outcomes and Challenges

Esophageal Surgery Esophagectomy remains the cornerstone of curative-intent therapy for resectable EC. However, it is associated with substantial perioperative morbidity (30–60%) and mortality (2–10%), especially in older adults. Retrospective and population-based studies consistently show that patients aged ≥70 or ≥ 75 years are at increased risk for:

- Postoperative cardiac and pulmonary complications, including atrial fibrillation, pneumonia, and acute respiratory distress syndrome (ARDS).
- Longer hospital stays and higher rates of non-home discharge.
- Increased 30-day and 90-day mortality, particularly in frail or comorbid patients.
- Higher costs of care and resource utilization, driven by complication management and prolonged recovery.

Importantly, long-term overall survival (OS) and disease-free survival (DFS) tend to be lower in elderly patients, though cancer-specific survival (CSS) may remain comparable to younger cohorts. This suggests that non-cancer-related mortality—rather than tumor progression—is the primary driver of inferior OS in this group.

Gastric Surgery Surgical resection remains the cornerstone of curative treatment for resectable GC. However, outcomes in elderly patients vary considerably depending on physiological status, comorbidities, tumor burden, and surgical approach.

Data from retrospective cohort studies reveal that elderly patients have higher rates of ASA class III or IV and a greater prevalence of cardiovascular and pulmonary diseases. Despite these challenges, surgical morbidity—particularly technical complications such as anastomotic leakage or intra-abdominal abscess—are not significantly higher in older patients when modern techniques and perioperative protocols are applied. In contrast, medical complications, particularly pneumonia and cardiac events, are markedly more frequent.

Interestingly, elderly patients often undergo shorter operations and experience less intraoperative blood loss, possibly due to less aggressive surgical approaches, including limited lymphadenectomy. Despite this, the curative intent of surgery remains intact, and CSS is preserved. Length of hospital stay and in-hospital mortality are increased in older patients, likely reflecting their reduced physiological reserve.

15.4.1 Minimally Invasive Surgery: A Viable Option for the Elderly

Esophageal Surgery Minimally invasive esophagectomy (MIE), encompassing thoracoscopic, laparoscopic, and robotic-assisted techniques, offers several key advantages over traditional open esophagectomy (OE). These benefits include:

- Reduced intraoperative blood loss.
- Lower rates of pulmonary complications.
- Shorter hospital stays.
- Faster functional recovery.
- Reduced postoperative pain.
- Improved lymph node retrieval compared with open approaches.
- Lower postoperative inflammatory response.
- Better tolerance of adjuvant therapy due to reduced surgical stress.

Studies have shown that when performed by experienced teams in high-volume centers, MIE achieves oncologic outcomes comparable to OE (clear margin [R0] resection rates, lymph node yields, and survival). Compared with open surgery, MIE is associated with lower pulmonary morbidity (20–25% versus 35–40%), reduced intraoperative blood loss (200–300 mL versus 400–600 mL), shorter intensive care unit stays (2–3 versus 5–6 days), and faster postoperative recovery [1, 2]. A meta-analysis by Markar et al. demonstrated that older patients undergoing open esophagectomy had significantly higher in-hospital mortality (8–10% versus 3–5% in younger patients) and increased pulmonary complications (up to 40% versus 25%) [1, 4]. In contrast, studies of MIE have reported comparable 30-day mortality between elderly and younger patients (1.5–2% versus 1–2%) and similar anastomotic leak rates (~6–7%) [2, 3, 5].

Thoracoscopic esophagectomy (TE) in patients aged ≥75 years has achieved acceptable outcomes, with in-hospital mortality as low as 4% and pulmonary complication rates of 20–25% [2]. However, pulmonary complications independently predict poorer survival in elderly cohorts, with hazard ratios of 3.51 for OS and 3.08 for recurrence-free survival (RFS) [2]. Five-year survival in octogenarians after OE remains lower (20–25%) than in younger groups (~35–40%), but MIE appears to mitigate this decline, achieving outcomes closer to those of non-elderly patients [3, 5].

Robotic-assisted Ivor Lewis esophagectomy (RAIL) has further enhanced surgical precision. In the largest series involving elderly patients, RAIL achieved 100% R0 resection, a mean lymph node yield of 20–21, and no 30-day mortality [9]. Overall complication rates were 26.9%, decreasing to 19% after the learning curve was surpassed, with pulmonary morbidity reduced compared with open surgery [9]. Operative time decreased significantly after the first 20 cases (514 versus 397 min, $p < 0.005$) [9]. Stratification by age revealed no significant differences in severe complications, although elderly patients had higher rates of cardiac arrhythmias (12–15% versus 5–7%) [9].

Gastric Surgery Minimally invasive gastrectomy (MIG), encompassing both laparoscopic and robotic-assisted approaches, is increasingly adopted for the management of GC in elderly patients. It is associated with several advantages:

- Reduced intraoperative blood loss.
- Fewer postoperative complications.
- Faster return of gastrointestinal function.
- Shorter hospital stays.
- Improved QoL compared to open gastrectomy (OG).

Numerous meta-analyses demonstrate that MIG is associated with substantially reduced intraoperative blood loss (120–150 mL versus 250–300 mL for OG), lower overall complication rates (18–22% versus 28–35%), faster recovery of bowel function (3–4 versus 5–6 days), and shorter hospital stays (9–11 versus 13–15 days) [12–15]. Operative time is generally longer, but this prolongation diminishes with surgical experience and does not adversely affect perioperative outcomes [12, 15].

Critically, MIG does not compromise oncological adequacy: mean lymph node retrieval (28–32 nodes) and R0 resection rates (>95%) are comparable to those achieved with OG [12–14]. Propensity-matched analyses have reported equivalent 5-year OS between MIG and OG, with some studies indicating marginally improved survival in laparoscopic cohorts, likely reflecting selection of earlier-stage disease [12–14]. In elderly patients, the reduced physiological stress of MIG facilitates enhanced postoperative recovery and greater tolerance of adjuvant therapy, which may translate into improved long-term outcomes. Among stage II–III patients, the lower morbidity associated with MIG supports better adherence to adjuvant chemotherapy, a factor consistently linked to improved survival [12, 13].

For example, in studies analyzing cohorts of octogenarians, overall complication rates remain elevated (30–35%), with cardiopulmonary events particularly prevalent (15–20% versus 8–10% in younger patients) [14, 15]. Nevertheless, the minimally invasive approach significantly reduces operative trauma and perioperative mortality relative to OG, with in-hospital mortality rates reported at 2–3% for MIG compared with 5–6% for OG [12, 14, 15]. DFS appears consistent across age groups, indicating preserved cancer control, whereas OS is influenced predominantly by comorbidities and frailty rather than surgical modality [16–18].

15.5 Multimodal Therapy in the Elderly: Underutilization and Potential

Esophageal Cancer Neoadjuvant chemoradiotherapy (nCRT) followed by surgery is the standard of care for locally advanced EC, yet elderly patients are frequently excluded from trials and often undertreated in clinical practice. Barriers to multimodal therapy include concerns about:

- Increased toxicity, particularly with platinum-based regimens.
- Decreased completion rates of therapy.
- Increased risk of postoperative morbidity after neoadjuvant treatment.

Despite these concerns, data suggest that fit elderly patients may tolerate nCRT with acceptable toxicity and derive survival benefits, particularly in cases of advanced-stage adenocarcinoma. Strategies to optimize tolerance include:

- Use of modified chemotherapy regimens, such as oral S-1 instead of platinum-doublets.
- Involved-field irradiation (IFI) rather than elective nodal irradiation to minimize toxicity.
- Tailored dose adjustments based on renal function and nutritional status.

Definitive chemoradiotherapy (dCRT) remains a viable non-surgical option for patients unfit for surgery. It has shown favorable outcomes, particularly in squamous cell carcinoma, with acceptable toxicity when using modern radiation techniques and geriatric-adapted chemotherapy.

Gastric Cancer Adjuvant and neoadjuvant therapies are underutilized in elderly patients, often due to concerns about toxicity and tolerability. Nonetheless, select patients with good performance status may benefit from perioperative chemotherapy or adjuvant chemoradiotherapy. Trials such as ACTS-GC and MAGIC have established the efficacy of multimodal approaches; however, data specific to patients aged ≥75 remain limited.

Emerging regimens with reduced toxicity profiles (e.g., S-1 monotherapy) may be better suited for older patients. Prospective studies evaluating geriatric-specific outcomes, including QoL, treatment adherence, and functional recovery, are urgently needed.

15.6 Conclusion and Future Perspectives

Esophageal Surgery With a rapidly aging global population, the management of EC in elderly patients is an emerging priority in surgical oncology. Although advanced age is associated with increased perioperative risk, age alone should not preclude curative treatment. CGA, frailty evaluation, and personalized treatment planning are essential to ensure optimal outcomes.

Minimally invasive surgical techniques, tailored chemotherapy regimens, and individualized radiation protocols represent pivotal strategies to reduce toxicity while maintaining oncologic efficacy. Elderly patients with good performance status can safely undergo esophagectomy, particularly when treated at specialized centers with multidisciplinary expertise.

Future research must focus on conducting prospective trials including elderly patients, with stratification by frailty rather than age alone, integrating QoL and functional outcomes into treatment endpoints, and developing geriatric-informed guidelines for EC management.

Ultimately, a paradigm shift toward personalized, frailty-adapted care will be critical to improving survival and maintaining dignity and QoL in elderly patients with EC.

Gastric Cancer GC in the elderly is a growing clinical challenge due to demographic shifts and the complex interplay of frailty, comorbidity, and tumor biology. Surgical intervention remains the mainstay of treatment for resectable disease, even in patients aged 80 and above. However, frailty assessment and individualized risk stratification are essential to guide therapeutic decisions.

Minimally invasive approaches, appropriate lymphadenectomy, and judicious use of multimodal therapies can optimize outcomes in fit elderly patients. Conversely, in those with significant physiological impairment, less aggressive but tailored strategies may preserve QoL without compromising palliation.

Future research should focus on integrating frailty metrics into surgical and oncological trials, standardizing preoperative assessment protocols, and evaluating patient-centered outcomes such as QoL and functional independence.

Multidisciplinary care models, incorporating geriatric expertise, are key to addressing the nuanced needs of this expanding patient population.

References

1. Baranov NS, Slootmans C, van Workum F, et al. Outcomes of curative esophageal cancer surgery in elderly: a meta-analysis. World J Gastrointest Oncol. 2021;13(2):131–46.
2. Kuwabara S, Kobayashi K, Sudo N. Outcomes of elderly patients following thoracoscopic esophagectomy for esophageal cancer. Langenbeck's Arch Surg. 2023;408(1):56.
3. Baranov NS, van Workum F, van der Maas J, et al. Influence of age on complications and overall survival after Ivor Lewis totally minimally invasive esophagectomy. J Gastrointest Surg. 2019;23(7):1293–300.
4. Schlottmann F, Strassle PD, Nayyar A, et al. Postoperative outcomes of esophagectomy for cancer in elderly patients. J Surg Res. 2018;229:9–14.
5. Aoyama T, Hara K, Kazama K, et al. The short- and long-term outcomes of esophagectomy for esophageal cancer in patients older than 75 years. Anticancer Res. 2020;40(2):1087–93.
6. Mantziari S, Teixeira Farinha H, Bouygues V, et al. Esophageal cancer in elderly patients, current treatment options and outcomes; a systematic review and pooled analysis. Cancers (Basel). 2021;13(9):2104.
7. Sugita Y, Nakamura T, Sawada R, et al. Safety and feasibility of minimally invasive esophagectomy for elderly esophageal cancer patients. Dis Esophagus. 2021;34(3):doaa083.
8. Moletta L, Pierobon ES, Capovilla G, et al. Short- and long-term outcomes in elderly patients with resectable esophageal cancer: upfront esophagectomy compared to surgery after neoadjuvant treatments. J Clin Med. 2024;13(14):4271.
9. Abbott A, Shridhar R, Hoffe S, et al. Robotic assisted Ivor Lewis esophagectomy in the elderly patient. J Gastrointest Oncol. 2015;6(1):31–8.
10. Yao J, Zhao X, Chen J, et al. Treatment strategies for elderly patients with locally advanced esophageal cancer: a systematic review and meta-analysis. BMC Cancer. 2024;24(1):1101.
11. Laurent A, Marechal R, Farinella E, et al. Esophageal cancer: outcome and potential benefit of esophagectomy in elderly patients. Thorac Cancer. 2022;13(19):2699–710.
12. Merga ZC, Lee JS, Gong CS. Outcomes of gastrectomy for gastric cancer in patients aged >80 years: a systematic literature review and meta-analysis. J Gastric Cancer. 2023;23(3):428–50.
13. Argillander TE, Festen S, van der Zaag-Loonen HJ, et al. Outcomes of surgical treatment of non-metastatic gastric cancer in patients aged 70 and older: a systematic review and meta-analysis. Eur J Surg Oncol. 2022;48(9):1882–94.
14. Xu Y, Wang Y, Xi C, et al. Is it safe to perform gastrectomy in gastric cancer patients aged 80 or older?: a meta-analysis and systematic review. Medicine (Baltimore). 2019;98(24):e16092.
15. He F, Xiong J, Liu H, et al. Laparoscopic gastrectomy versus open gastrectomy for gastric cancer in patients among octogenarians: a meta-analysis. Clin Transl Oncol. 2025;27(2):593–603.
16. Tang WZ, Tan ZK, Qiu LY, et al. Prevalence and unfavorable outcome of frailty in older adults with gastric cancer: a systematic review and meta-analysis. Support Care Cancer. 2024;32(2):115.
17. Saif MW, Makrilia N, Zalonis A, et al. Gastric cancer in the elderly: an overview. Eur J Surg Oncol. 2010;36(8):709–17.
18. Zhao B, Zhang S, Chen Y, et al. Risk factors for preoperative frailty in older patients with gastric cancer: a systematic review and meta-analysis. Support Care Cancer. 2024;32(7):450.

Colon Surgery

16

Paolo Sapienza, Daniele Crocetti, Michelangelo Miccini, Immacolata Iannone, and Enrico Fiori

16.1 Introduction

Life expectancy is growing in the Western world, and some age-related diseases are likewise becoming more prevalent. The geriatric population represents one of the fastest-growing subsets of the U.S. population. By 2030, it is estimated that 20% of the total population will be older than 75 years. As the population ages, an increasing number of elderly patients will require colon surgery.

Colon cancer is one of the most common tumors in Western countries, ranking as the third most prevalent tumor among both sexes, following breast and lung neoplasms. It is the second leading cause of death, after lung cancer. Incidence and prevalence vary by country due to differing lifestyles and screening programs. In Italy, colon cancer is the second most common tumor and affects nearly 50,000 patients each year, and most of them are male patients.

The risk of colon cancer increases with age, and population aging, along with the decline of other causes of death such as cardiovascular diseases, contributes to a higher prevalence of colon cancer in the elderly.

This presents a significant challenge for Western healthcare systems because various factors related to aging, such as frailty and comorbidities, affect decision-making, particularly as the algorithms for colon cancer treatment become more complex with age.

The risk of delaying surgery because of difficulties accessing the public hospital is crucial in the attempt to cure elderly patients. Although our health system is universalistic, accessing the screening program can be extremely complex for the elderly, and referral to private facilities may be impossible due to economic difficulties.

P. Sapienza (✉) · D. Crocetti · M. Miccini · I. Iannone · E. Fiori
Department of Surgery, Sapienza University of Rome, Rome, Italy
e-mail: paolo.sapienza@uniroma1.it; daniele.crocetti@uniroma1.it; michelangelo.miccini@uniroma1.it; immacolata.iannone@uniroma1.it; enrico.fiori@uniroma1.it

P. Carcoforo, F. Catena (eds.), *Geriatric Surgery*, Updates in Surgery,
https://doi.org/10.1007/978-3-032-24281-5_16

16.2 Preoperative Geriatric Assessment

The variability in aging presentations impacts the distinction between chronological and physiological age, affecting patients' access to and continuity of care, and thus influencing the integration of geriatric tools in the decision-making process.

Geriatric Assessment (GA) should theoretically enable the identification of functional status, comorbidities, social and economic circumstances, mental condition, emotional state, nutritional health, polypharmacy therapy, mobility, cognition, and geriatric syndromes.

The prevalence of frailty in the geriatric population reaches 40%, thus determining poor survival rates and a great number of postoperative complications. Consequently, frail[1] patients require more attention and care, as they are less able to handle stressful situations, i.e., surgery or chemotherapy. Frail patients develop a higher incidence of complications and a poorer tolerance to cytostatic therapy.

However, the heterogeneity of the geriatric population affected by colon cancer emphasizes the need for preoperative assessment to provide tailored treatment and enhance postoperative outcomes. Some clinicians involved in the care of geriatric patients have adopted the GA to detect the geriatric domain impairments and identify patients at increased risk for adverse outcomes who might benefit from an intervention. However, the domains included in a GA vary significantly across studies of geriatric patients, and there is still no consensus on which items or screening tools should be used to evaluate these domains.

Performing a full GA on all geriatric surgical patients is too time-consuming for clinical practice. It may be unnecessary because most patients can be considered fit for surgery. Researchers have focused on the predictive ability and clinical value of separate domains of a GA and related easy-to-administer screening tools to select those patients for whom a full GA might be indicated. Discrepancies in outcomes between these studies currently hamper the implementation of a preoperative geriatric assessment in clinical practice.

Synthetically, we recommend a routine assessment of nutritional and mental status before surgery in the elderly population, as preoperative optimization of these domains might significantly improve outcomes [1–3].

16.3 Delay in Colon Cancer Surgery

Delays in cancer treatment can adversely affect outcomes, creating challenges within health systems globally. The cornerstone of curative therapy for colon cancer is performing surgery within one month of diagnosis. Systematic reviews and a meta-analysis in the literature confirm that delays in diagnosis are linked to an increased risk of patients presenting with advanced stages of colon cancer. Typically,

[1] There is no one clear-cut definition of frailty used in clinical practice; the term captures the natural, highly individual, age-related decline in health and the resulting vulnerability associated with this.

any treatment for colon cancer should commence within two months of diagnosis at the latest, and ideally within one month [4]. A treatment delay of four weeks correlates with a higher risk of death. For surgery, this risk increases by 6–8% for every four-week delay. This effect is even more pronounced for certain radiotherapy and systemic indications, leading to a 13% increased risk of death for adjuvant systemic treatment for colon cancer [5].

We acknowledge that elderly patients may face multifactorial delays in treatment and might not start treatment until they are medically cleared for surgery and have completed all required preoperative evaluations. Nevertheless, we strongly support initiatives to minimize system-level delays by creating a dedicated channel within the diagnostic and therapeutic care pathways for geriatric patients dealing with colon cancer.

Another aspect to consider is that geriatric patients may face psychosocial and socioeconomic challenges. Regardless of prevalence, a cancer diagnosis is a stressful event for patients of all ages, often causing significant fear and uncertainty; therefore, symptoms of anxiety, depression, and other forms of psychological distress are hardly surprising. It is estimated that, overall, between 35% and 50% of cancer patients experience psychological issues, with adjustment disorder with depressed mood being the most common clinical diagnosis. Accurately identifying psychological distress is crucial for providing optimal care to individuals with colon cancer, as reducing psychological morbidity improves overall well-being and may even offer a slight survival advantage. Comorbid psychological conditions can affect treatment and recovery. Depressive symptoms can lead to increased pain and diminished physical and social functioning. Furthermore, depression can influence both the severity and number of side effects, contributing to heightened anxiety and fatigue experienced by cancer patients. Additionally, depressed patients tend to use medical services more often, incur higher healthcare costs, and have longer hospital stays than those without depression, placing an additional burden on the healthcare system. Given these potential consequences, any signs of psychological distress in elderly cancer patients should be addressed and managed effectively. Patients may express their emotional distress verbally or non-verbally. However, various barriers can hinder doctors' ability to detect their patients' distress. Patients may normalize or somatize their feelings or feel it is inappropriate to discuss them. Clinicians may lack the necessary skills and knowledge to recognize distress. Since anxiety and depression can mimic the physical symptoms of cancer or its treatments, this can further reduce the chances of detection.

16.4 Comprehensive Multidisciplinary Care Program

Despite significant progress in perioperative care, 30-day morbidity has not shown substantial improvement, with rates ranging from 19.7% to 37.4%. Reducing the risk of postoperative complications and functional decline remains essential. Surgery is a major stressor that causes a fourfold increase in major postoperative complications among the elderly. Conceptually, three strategies can help mitigate the impact of colon cancer surgery on elderly patients [6]. First, through prehabilitation—by optimizing functional capacity before surgery with exercise training, nutritional support, and management of comorbidities—patients become more resilient. Second, by minimizing surgical impact using minimally invasive techniques and enhanced recovery protocols, which reduce the perioperative stress response, tissue injury, and metabolic disturbance, potentially leading to fewer complications and less postoperative pain. Third, facilitating early discharge to a rehabilitation center counteracts the negative effects of prolonged hospital stays, such as low daily activity, and decreases the risk of hospital-acquired infections. Through rehabilitation, the goal is to restore preoperative function, thereby decreasing vulnerability to other illnesses and improving the patient's quality of life.

16.5 Prehabilitation

Functional capacity is a key factor affecting positive outcomes after surgery. After a diagnosis of colon cancer, the period before surgery typically lasts several weeks—an ideal window for multimodal prehabilitation. Studies have shown that prehabilitation can lead to meaningful clinical improvements in a patient's preoperative condition and surgical results. Better cardiorespiratory fitness before surgery is thought to enhance physiological reserve and the patient's ability to cope with stress related to surgery. Furthermore, higher functional capacity is independently associated with a lower risk of postoperative complications in colon cancer patients. One main goal of prehabilitation is to improve functional capacity to support postoperative recovery. Three randomized clinical trials with similar multimodal prehabilitation programs were included in a recent Cochrane review [7]. We believe that a customized multimodal prehabilitation program [8] could also benefit elderly patients undergoing elective resection of non-metastasized colon cancer, aiming to reduce severe postoperative complications and promote better functional recovery. The specific approach needed for this should be explored through further randomized controlled trials. Currently, there is no specific program in the literature that is adaptable to all elderly patients, regardless of different risk factors or coexisting conditions. In conclusion, regular physical activity (such as walking for 30 min), smoking cessation, and immune-nutrition (e.g., a specially designed shake to support immune health) are essential. The latter aims to combat malnutrition and related complications following colon surgery.

16.6 Enhanced Recovery Care After Surgery

Enhanced Recovery care After Surgery (ERAS®) is a multidisciplinary care program aimed at promoting rapid recovery in patients. It is well established that following the components of the ERAS® protocol is linked to improved outcomes. ERAS® has become recognized as the gold standard of care to manage patients undergoing colorectal surgery. Many studies have demonstrated that ERAS® is safe, cost-effective, and shortens the length of hospital stay. Several studies have demonstrated a correlation between adherence to the components of the ERAS® and superior outcomes. However, elderly patients have higher levels of comorbidity, frailty and social care requirements. Therefore, the elderly need specific ERAS® strategies to optimize the length of recovery and to reduce postoperative complications and their sequelae [9]. Probably, not all elderly patients can comply with the components of an ERAS® program, and benefit from it to the same extent as younger patients. Future investigations should be focused on older patients with comorbidities to better define the specific borders of ERAS® in this subset of patients.

16.7 Surgical Operation and Technical Aspects

The choice of surgical procedures and the use of minimally invasive surgery (MIS) are essential for safely performing operations on elderly patients. MIS offers benefits over open surgery, such as smaller incisions, less pain, faster recovery of eating, a lower rate of postoperative complications, and shorter hospital stays. In addition to favorable short-term outcomes, the long-term results of MIS are comparable to those of open surgery. Therefore, MIS is a preferred alternative to open surgery when performed by surgeons properly trained in this specific technique. Due to its minimally invasive nature, MIS appears especially suitable for elderly patients.

However, the surgical technique remains unchanged regardless of the patient's age. Several key technical aspects must be followed: the minimum acceptable free margin, distal to the lower edge of the tumor, should be at least 5 cm. In right or transverse colonic resections, the ileocolic, right colic, or middle colic vessels at the root of the mesocolon should be ligated. Removing the apical lymph nodes allows for a more accurate prognostic assessment. Specifically, in cases of right colon and hepatic flexure colon cancer, a right hemicolectomy with ligation of the origin of the ileocolic, right colic, and right branch of the middle colic vascular pedicles is indicated. The role of complete mesocolic excision with central venous ligation—which involves extending lymph node dissection up to the right lateral margin of the superior mesenteric artery—remains debated; this approach could be considered for locally advanced right colon tumors. Furthermore, in cases of transverse colon cancer, resection of the transverse colon with ligation of the middle colonic pedicle can be performed. Alternatively, a right hemicolectomy extended to the transverse colon, with creation of a distal ileo-transverse or ileo-descending anastomosis, may be considered: this results in a higher number of lymph nodes recovered, a lower risk of anastomotic dehiscence, and similar survival rates. Extended right hemicolectomy, left hemicolectomy, or segmental resection of the splenic flexure can be performed when tumors involve the splenic flexure of the colon; in fact, there are no statistically significant differences in complication rates or survival. In left colon resections, the left colic and sigmoid pedicles should be ligated, and a corresponding lymphadenectomy should be carried out. In sigmoid resections, ligating the inferior mesenteric artery after its origin from the left colic artery is considered sufficient to achieve radicality. For tumors in the descending colon: perform a left hemicolectomy with ligation of the left colonic and sigmoid vascular pedicles, followed by intraperitoneal colorectal anastomosis.

We should also consider that in right colon neoplasms, standard lymphadenectomy should include the ileocolic lymph nodes and those from the right branch of the middle colic. For left colon and sigmoid cancers, the lymph nodes at the root of the inferior mesenteric artery should be included. Recent evidence indicates the oncological benefit of completely excising the mesocolon with standard central vascular ligation during right hemicolectomy, which involves ligating the ileocolic vessels at their origin by preparing the superior mesenteric vein. However, this method has not yet been validated by rigorous meta-analyses and is also linked to potentially serious complications. MIS should theoretically be preferred over an open approach in the elderly population; however, current literature [10–12] lacks studies offering a comprehensive evaluation of video-laparoscopic, robotic-assisted, or open surgery by comparing perioperative and long-term outcomes for patients with colon cancer. Present studies suggest that robotic surgery is associated with longer operative times but shorter hospital stays compared to laparoscopic surgery. Conversion rates are significantly higher in laparoscopic procedures. While no significant differences are typically found in anastomotic leak rates, the robotic approach yields a higher number of lymph nodes, less estimated blood loss, and earlier bowel canalization. A specific study on octogenarians and nonagenarians indicated that robotic surgery is linked to a significantly shorter length of stay but higher total hospital costs compared to laparoscopic surgery. Other short-term outcomes for this population were similar between the two procedures, including in-hospital mortality, perioperative complications, and unfavorable discharge. In conclusion, we suggest a robotic approach for colon cancer whenever possible in elderly patients.

16.8 Postoperative Care

We should recognize that an increasing number of studies highlight the importance of nontraditional risk factors in adherence to adjuvant chemotherapy, especially among elderly patients. Low income, psychiatric illness, or cognitive impairment can significantly impact adherence. The factors that hinder postoperative care compliance are not fully understood but include age, sex, race, ethnicity, marital status, socioeconomic status, patient choice, and related health conditions. While many of these factors are clinical, non-clinical factors also influence adherence and are linked to the patient care experience, particularly patient-provider communication and the therapeutic relationship. Current research [13] shows that effective patient-centered communication promotes engagement, trust, and understanding. This type of communication has been shown to improve the ability to discuss difficult clinical topics and strengthen patient-provider relationships. It also fosters engagement, trust, and understanding. Such communication has been demonstrated to improve treatment adherence in primary care and various illnesses; however, further research is necessary to understand this relationship among colon cancer patients and to identify multiple intervention points, especially in subgroups with high rates of non-adherence to adjuvant therapy. In conclusion, we recommend a comprehensive investigation of all potential causes that may delay or prevent the initiation of additional adjuvant therapy in elderly patients.

References

1. Huisman MG, Kok M, de Bock GH, van Leeuwen BL. Delivering tailored surgery to older cancer patients: preoperative geriatric assessment domains and screening tools – a systematic review of systematic reviews. Eur J Surg Oncol. 2017;43(1):1–14.
2. Teraishi F, Yoshida Y, Shoji R, et al. Subjective global assessment for nutritional screening and its impact on surgical outcomes: a prospective study in older patients with colorectal cancer. Langenbecks Arch Surg. 2024;409(1):356.
3. Tsai CY, Liu KH, Lai CC, et al. Association of preoperative frailty and postoperative delirium in older cancer patients undergoing elective abdominal surgery: a prospective observational study in Taiwan. Biomed J. 2023;46(4):100557.
4. Tørring ML, Murchie P, Hamilton W, et al. Evidence of advanced stage colorectal cancer with longer diagnostic intervals: a pooled analysis of seven primary care cohorts comprising 11 720 patients in five countries. Br J Cancer. 2017;117(6):888–97.
5. Hanna TP, King WD, Thibodeau S, et al. Mortality due to cancer treatment delay: systematic review and meta-analysis. BMJ. 2020;371:m4087.
6. Souwer ETD, Bastiaannet E, de Bruijn S, et al. Comprehensive multidisciplinary care program for elderly colorectal cancer patients: "from prehabilitation to independence". Eur J Surg Oncol. 2018;44(12):1894–900.
7. Molenaar CJ, van Rooijen SJ, Fokkenrood HJ, et al. Prehabilitation versus no prehabilitation to improve functional capacity, reduce postoperative complications and improve quality of life in colorectal cancer surgery. Cochrane Database Syst Rev. 2022;5(5):CD013259.
8. Molenaar CJL, Minnella EM, Coca-Martinez M, et al. Effect of multimodal prehabilitation on reducing postoperative complications and enhancing functional capacity following colorectal cancer surgery: the PREHAB randomized clinical trial. JAMA Surg. 2023;158(6):572–81.
9. Bagnall NM, Malietzis G, Kennedy RH, et al. A systematic review of enhanced recovery care after colorectal surgery in elderly patients. Colorectal Dis. 2014;16(12):947–56.
10. Negrut RL, Cote A, Caus VA, Maghiar AM. Systematic review and meta-analysis of laparoscopic versus robotic-assisted surgery for colon cancer: efficacy, safety, and outcomes – a focus on studies from 2020–2024. Cancers (Basel). 2024;16(8):1552.
11. Feng Q, Yuan W, Li T, et al. Robotic versus laparoscopic surgery for middle and low rectal cancer (REAL): short-term outcomes of a multicentre randomised controlled trial. Lancet Gastroenterol Hepatol. 2022;7(11):991–1004.
12. Lu CC, Lu CT, Chang KY, et al. Robot-assisted vs. laparoscopic right hemicolectomy in octogenarians and nonagenarians: an analysis of the US nationwide inpatient sample 2005–2018. Aging Clin Exp Res. 2024;36(1):193.
13. Mitchell KR, Boyle JR, Juricekova L, Brown RF. Adjuvant chemotherapy non-adherence, patient-centered communication, and patient-level factors in elderly breast and colon cancer patients. Cancer Med. 2023;12(10):11915–29.

17 Rectal Surgery

Gerardo Sarno, Giovanni Fabbrocile, Elio Donnarumma, Nicoletta Stolfi, Gennaro Cascone, Luisa Ambrosio, and Alessandro Puzziello

17.1 Introduction

Rectal surgery encompasses a wide spectrum of procedures aimed at treating diseases affecting the rectum, including benign conditions such as inflammatory bowel disease and rectal prolapse, as well as malignant diseases, predominantly rectal cancer. The rectum's unique anatomical location within the pelvis poses surgical challenges, necessitating precise techniques to achieve oncological clearance while preserving function.

Over recent decades, rectal surgery has evolved substantially. Traditional open surgery remains a cornerstone; however, minimally invasive approaches including laparoscopic and robotic-assisted techniques have gained prominence due to their potential to reduce morbidity, hasten recovery, and improve cosmetic outcomes. These advancements are particularly relevant in the context of rectal cancer, where total mesorectal excision (TME) is the standard surgical approach, aimed at achieving local disease control and improving survival [1, 2].

Patient selection and perioperative management have become increasingly personalized. Factors such as tumor staging, patient comorbidities, and anatomical considerations guide surgical planning. The role of neoadjuvant chemoradiotherapy has also expanded, aiming to downstage tumors and improve resectability [3].

A growing area of interest is the management of rectal cancer in elderly patients. This population often presents with distinct challenges, including reduced physiological reserve, multiple comorbidities, and increased frailty. Surgical decision-making in elderly patients requires balancing oncological efficacy with risks of

G. Sarno · G. Fabbrocile · E. Donnarumma · N. Stolfi · G. Cascone · L. Ambrosio · A. Puzziello (✉)
General Surgery and Transplantation Unit, San Giovanni di Dio e Ruggi D'Aragona University Hospital, Scuola Medica Salernitana, University of Salerno, Salerno, Italy
e-mail: gerardo.sarno@sangiovannieruggi.it; giovanni.fabbrocile@sangiovannieruggi.it; apuzziello@unisa.it

P. Carcoforo, F. Catena (eds.), *Geriatric Surgery*, Updates in Surgery,
https://doi.org/10.1007/978-3-032-24281-5_17

complications and quality of life [4, 5]. Recent systematic reviews have compared outcomes between elderly and non-elderly patients, noting differences in survival, complication rates, and postoperative recovery [6]. Personalized treatment paradigms, incorporating minimally invasive surgery and tailored perioperative care, are being developed to optimize outcomes in this demographic [7].

This chapter aims to provide a comprehensive overview of rectal surgery, focusing on surgical techniques, perioperative considerations, and patient outcomes, with a dedicated section on the elderly population. By synthesizing current evidence and clinical practices, the chapter intends to serve as a resource for surgeons, oncologists, and healthcare providers involved in rectal disease management.

17.2 Surgical Anatomy of the Rectum

The rectum is the distal part of the large intestine, extending from the sigmoid colon to the anal canal, and typically about 12–15 cm in length. Anatomically, it lies within the pelvis and is surrounded by critical structures that must be considered during surgical dissection. The upper third of the rectum is intraperitoneal, while the lower two-thirds are extraperitoneal. Laterally, the mesorectum contains lymphatic tissue, blood vessels, and fatty tissue, enclosed by the mesorectal fascia. Preservation of this fascial plane is crucial during TME, as it minimizes local recurrence and improves oncologic outcomes [8].

Anteriorly, the rectum is in proximity to the bladder, seminal vesicles, and prostate in males, and the vagina and uterus in females. The Denonvilliers' fascia separates the rectum from these anterior structures. Posteriorly lies the presacral fascia overlying the sacrum. Laterally, autonomic nerves—particularly the hypogastric nerves and the inferior hypogastric plexus—are responsible for urinary and sexual function. Surgical technique must aim to preserve these structures to reduce postoperative dysfunction.

The vascular supply of the rectum is primarily through the superior rectal artery (branch of the inferior mesenteric artery), with additional supply from the middle and inferior rectal arteries. Venous drainage involves the superior rectal vein (portal circulation) and the middle and inferior rectal veins (systemic circulation), contributing to the potential for hematogenous metastasis. Lymphatic drainage follows a predictable pattern, with upper rectal lesions draining along the superior rectal and inferior mesenteric nodes, and lower rectal lesions to internal iliac and inguinal nodes.

17.3 Surgical Approaches

Surgical technique in rectal surgery depends on tumor location, disease stage, patient anatomy, and institutional expertise especially when related to elderly patients (Table 17.1).

The following are the principal approaches.

Table 17.1 Surgical approaches and outcomes in rectal cancer in elderly patients

Study/ Author	Year	Study type	Population	Surgical approach	Main outcome
Manceau et al. [1]	2012	Systematic review	Elderly vs. non-elderly patients	Rectal resection	No significant difference in mortality or major complications
Spinelli et al. [2]	2017	Narrative review	Elderly with comorbidities	Personalized treatment	Need for tailored approaches based on frailty and functional status
Badic et al. [3]	2021	Retrospective study	Elderly patients with stage III–IV	Permanent ostomy	Higher ostomy prevalence; negative impact on survival
De Felice et al. [4]	2020	Review	Patients ≥70 with locally advanced rectal cancer	Chemoradiotherapy + surgery	Multidisciplinary assessment critical; selected patients benefit from treatment
Halfter et al. [5]	2023	Retrospective real-world	Elderly population	Mixed	Limited survival gains for elderly despite therapeutic advances
Huang CK [6]	2024	Review	Elderly patients with rectal cancer	Variable	Undertreatment common; Comprehensive Geriatric Assessment recommended
Zhang et al. [7]	2021	Retrospective cohort study	Patients ≥80 years	Laparoscopic vs. open	Laparoscopy showed fewer complications and shorter hospital stays
Mun et al. [8]	2025	Population-based cohort	Patients ≥70 years	Radical surgery + adjuvant therapy	Improved survival with curative surgery and chemotherapy
Abir et al. [9]	2004	Review	Elderly patients	Variable	Age alone should not determine treatment strategy
Pulvirenti et al. [10]	2025	Multicenter cohort study	Elderly patients with locally advanced rectal cancer	Neoadjuvant chemoradiotherapy + surgery	Good oncologic outcomes in selected elderly patients
Horsey et al. [11]	2022	National database study	Elderly patients	Robotic, laparoscopic, open	Robotic and laparoscopic approaches yielded better short- and long-term outcomes

17.3.1 Open Surgery

Traditional open rectal surgery remains an important option, especially in complex cases such as locally advanced tumors, prior abdominal surgery, or where minimally invasive options are not feasible. Open surgery offers tactile feedback and broad access but is associated with higher postoperative pain, longer recovery, and greater blood loss compared to laparoscopic approaches [9].

17.3.2 Laparoscopic Surgery

Laparoscopic rectal resection has been shown to offer similar oncologic outcomes to open surgery in multiple randomized controlled trials and meta-analyses, with advantages including reduced postoperative pain, faster return of bowel function, lower wound complication rates, and shorter hospital stays [10, 11]. Challenges include limited visualization and maneuverability within the deep pelvis, especially in obese patients or those with narrow pelvic anatomy. Nonetheless, it is now considered standard of care in many centers.

In elderly patients, laparoscopic surgery has demonstrated favorable outcomes. A large retrospective cohort of patients aged ≥80 showed reduced complication rates, blood loss, and faster recovery compared to open surgery, with no significant difference in long-term survival [12].

17.3.3 Robotic-Assisted Surgery

Robotic surgery addresses some of the limitations of laparoscopy by offering improved ergonomics, three-dimensional visualization, and articulated instruments. It allows for precise dissection in confined pelvic spaces, making it particularly advantageous for low rectal tumors. Several studies have shown comparable oncologic outcomes to laparoscopy and potential advantages in terms of lower conversion rates and better preservation of autonomic nerves [13].

A meta-analysis comparing robotic rectal resection outcomes in elderly vs. non-elderly patients found no significant difference in distal margins, lymph node yield, or postoperative complications, suggesting that robotic surgery is a safe option across age groups [6].

17.3.4 Transanal Approaches

Transanal minimally invasive surgery (TAMIS) and transanal total mesorectal excision (TaTME) are newer techniques that allow distal-to-proximal dissection from the anal canal. These techniques are particularly useful in patients with low rectal tumors where sphincter preservation is desired. TaTME has shown promising oncologic outcomes but requires significant technical expertise and has been associated with unique complications such as urethral injury [14].

17.4 Neoadjuvant and Adjuvant Therapy

Neoadjuvant chemoradiotherapy (CRT) is standard for locally advanced rectal cancer (T3–T4 or N+), aiming to reduce tumor size, downstage the disease, and increase the chance of sphincter-sparing surgery. The typical regimen involves long-course CRT with fluoropyrimidine-based chemotherapy and pelvic radiation (45–50.4 Gy). Alternatively, short-course radiotherapy (5 × 5 Gy) followed by delayed surgery may be used.

Evidence suggests that preoperative CRT leads to better local control compared to postoperative therapy. Pathological complete response (pCR) is achieved in approximately 15–20% of patients, and these individuals may be candidates for organ-preserving strategies under watch-and-wait protocols [15].

Postoperative (adjuvant) chemotherapy is typically considered in patients with pathologic stage III disease, particularly if no neoadjuvant treatment was given. Elderly patients, however, are less likely to receive adjuvant therapy due to concerns about tolerance and comorbidities [4, 16].

17.5 Perioperative Management

Enhanced Recovery After Surgery (ERAS®) protocols have become the standard in rectal surgery. These evidence-based pathways aim to reduce perioperative stress, shorten hospital stay, and improve outcomes. Key components include preoperative counseling, avoidance of mechanical bowel preparation when appropriate, carbohydrate loading, multimodal analgesia, early feeding, and mobilization.

In elderly patients, Comprehensive Geriatric Assessment (CGA) can help predict postoperative outcomes and identify modifiable risk factors. Studies have shown that frailty, rather than age alone, is the most significant predictor of postoperative morbidity and mortality [17].

Prehabilitation programs, including exercise, nutrition, and psychological support, are increasingly used to improve patient fitness before surgery. In rectal cancer patients undergoing neoadjuvant therapy, prehabilitation during the waiting period can mitigate treatment-related deconditioning [18].

17.6 Oncologic and Functional Outcomes

17.6.1 Oncologic Outcomes

Successful rectal cancer surgery is measured by clear resection margins (both circumferential and distal), adequate lymph node harvest (≥12 nodes), and minimization of local recurrence. TME has dramatically improved local control. The use of MRI to assess the circumferential resection margins (CRM) preoperatively allows surgeons to plan resections that reduce the risk of involved margins [19].

Minimally invasive approaches (laparoscopic and robotic) have consistently shown equivalent oncologic outcomes to open surgery in terms of CRM positivity, lymph node retrieval, and long-term survival [20]. Robotic surgery may offer a slight edge in very low rectal tumors due to improved pelvic access [13].

17.6.2 Functional Outcomes

Preservation of bowel, urinary, and sexual function is essential, especially for low anterior resection. Bowel dysfunction postoperatively may include urgency, frequency, clustering, and fecal incontinence—collectively referred to as low anterior resection syndrome (LARS). Nerve-sparing techniques are critical to reducing postoperative urinary and sexual dysfunction.

In elderly patients, these issues may be more pronounced due to baseline sphincter weakness and comorbid conditions. Ostomy creation (permanent or temporary) is more frequent in older populations, either due to technical challenges or concerns about recovery from anastomotic leak [21].

17.7 Elderly Patients in Rectal Surgery

The aging population has led to an increased incidence of rectal cancer among elderly individuals, with over 40% of new diagnoses occurring in patients aged 70 years and older. While chronological age alone should not preclude surgical treatment, physiological reserve, comorbidities, and functional status are critical in determining the optimal therapeutic approach.

17.7.1 Surgical Outcomes in the Elderly

Elderly patients undergoing rectal surgery have historically been perceived as high risk. However, multiple studies have demonstrated that with appropriate patient selection and perioperative optimization, outcomes can be comparable to those in younger cohorts. A systematic review comparing outcomes between elderly ($\geq$70 years) and non-elderly patients found no significant difference in mortality or major complications following surgery for rectal cancer [1]. However, elderly patients were less likely to receive neoadjuvant therapy and more likely to undergo a permanent stoma [2].

Laparoscopic and robotic approaches are particularly beneficial in elderly patients due to reduced operative trauma, lower rates of respiratory complications, and faster mobilization. A retrospective analysis of patients aged $\geq$80 undergoing laparoscopic resection showed significantly reduced postoperative complications, length of stay, and improved short-term outcomes compared to open surgery [12].

Despite this, elderly patients often experience disparities in treatment. A population-based study revealed lower rates of curative surgery and adjuvant chemotherapy in patients aged ≥75, even when controlling for disease stage and performance status [3, 4].

17.7.2 Ostomy and Quality of Life

The prevalence of permanent ostomy is higher in elderly patients, either due to technical difficulty in performing a safe anastomosis or a higher perceived risk of anastomotic leak. A large database study found that elderly patients with stage III–IV rectal cancer were more likely to receive a permanent stoma, with survival rates negatively impacted when compared to those who underwent anastomosis [5].

Despite concerns, studies indicate that many elderly patients adapt well to ostomies and report satisfactory quality of life. The key is proper preoperative counseling, patient education, and postoperative support from stoma care teams.

17.7.3 Personalized Treatment Approaches

Personalized care models, which consider frailty, comorbid conditions, cognitive function, and social support, are increasingly advocated for elderly rectal cancer patients. CGA has been shown to predict postoperative morbidity and guide decision-making [6].

In some cases, less aggressive treatment—including local excision or even non-operative management (watch-and-wait)—may be appropriate for frail patients achieving a clinical complete response after neoadjuvant therapy. While these approaches are still under investigation, they offer an alternative pathway for those unfit for major resection [7].

17.8 Conclusions

Rectal surgery is a dynamic field that integrates evolving surgical techniques, oncologic principles, and personalized patient care. Minimally invasive methods, including laparoscopic and robotic-assisted procedures, have become the standard for many patients, offering equivalent oncologic outcomes with reduced morbidity.

For elderly patients, surgical treatment must be approached with nuanced understanding. While age alone is not a contraindication, careful evaluation using geriatric assessment tools ensures optimal outcomes. Treatment should be individualized, balancing curative intent with functional preservation and patient preference.

Future directions in rectal surgery involve increasing the precision of surgical approaches, expanding organ-preserving strategies, and integrating molecular profiling for personalized oncology. Multidisciplinary care, supported by real-world evidence and clinical trials, remains the cornerstone of successful outcomes in both younger and elderly populations.

References

1. Manceau G, Karoui M, Werner A, et al. Comparative outcomes of rectal cancer surgery between elderly and non-elderly patients: a systematic review. Lancet Oncol. 2012;13(12):e525–36.
2. Spinelli A, Montroni I. Personalized treatments for elderly patients affected by rectal cancer. Colorectal Dis. 2017;19(10):879–80.
3. Badic B, Oguer M, Cariou M, et al. Ostomy prevalence and survival in elderly patients with stage III and IV rectal cancer. Geriatr Gerontol Int. 2021;21(8):670–5.
4. De Felice F, Crocetti D, Maiuri V, et al. Locally advanced rectal cancer: treatment approach in elderly patients. Curr Treat Options Oncol. 2020;21(1):1.
5. Halfter K, Schubert-Fritschle G, Röder F, et al. Advances in rectal cancer: real-world evidence suggests limited gains in prognosis for elderly patients. Cancer Epidemiol. 2023;86:102440.
6. Huang CK, Shih CH, Kao YS. Elderly rectal cancer: an updated review. Curr Oncol Rep. 2024;26(2):181–90.
7. Zhang Q, Liang J, Chen J, et al. Outcomes of laparoscopic versus open surgery in elderly patients with rectal cancer. Asian Pac J Cancer Prev. 2021;22(4):1325–9.
8. Mun JY, Han K, Yoo N, et al. Overall survival following radical surgery and postoperative chemotherapy in colorectal cancer patients aged ≥70 years: a population-based retrospective cohort study. BMC Cancer. 2025;25(1):1413.
9. Abir F, Alva S, Longo WE. The management of rectal cancer in the elderly. Surg Oncol. 2004;13(4):223–34.
10. Pulvirenti A, Parati C, Deidda S, et al. Textbook oncologic outcomes in elderly patients undergoing neoadjuvant chemoradiotherapy and surgery for locally advanced rectal cancer: a multicenter study. Updates Surg. 2025;77(8):2285–91.
11. Horsey ML, Parascandola SA, Sparks AD, et al. The impact of surgical approach on short- and long-term outcomes after rectal cancer resection in elderly patients: a national cancer database propensity score matched comparison of robotic, laparoscopic, and open approaches. Surg Endosc. 2022;36(2):1269–77.
12. Braga M, Pecorelli N, Ferrari D, et al. Results of 100 consecutive laparoscopic distal pancreatectomies: postoperative outcome, cost-benefit analysis, and quality of life assessment. Surg Endosc. 2015;29(7):1871–8.
13. Matsuyama T, Kinugasa Y, Nakajima Y, Kojima K. Robotic-assisted surgery for rectal cancer: Current state and future perspective. Ann Gastroenterol Surg. 2018;2(6):406–12.
14. Vignali A, Elmore U, Milone M, Rosati R. Transanal total mesorectal excision (TaTME): current status and future perspectives. Updates Surg. 2019;71(1):29–37.
15. Fokas E, Liersch T, Fietkau R, et al. Tumor regression grading after preoperative chemoradiotherapy for locally advanced rectal carcinoma revisited: updated results of the CAO/ARO/AIO-94 trial. J Clin Oncol. 2014;32(15):1554–62.
16. Bojer AS, Roikjær O. Elderly patients with colorectal cancer are oncologically undertreated. Eur J Surg Oncol. 2015;41(3):421–5.
17. Partridge JS, Harari D, Dhesi JK. Frailty in the older surgical patient: a review. Age Ageing. 2012;41(2):142–7.
18. Zhang X, Wang S, Ji W, et al. The effect of prehabilitation on the postoperative outcomes of patients undergoing colorectal surgery: a systematic review and meta-analysis. Front Oncol. 2022;12:958261.
19. Brown G, et al. Preoperative assessment of prognostic factors in rectal cancer using high-resolution magnetic resonance imaging. Br J Surg. 2003;90(3):355–64.
20. Bonjer HJ, Deijen CL, Haglind E, COLOR II Study Group. A randomized trial of laparoscopic versus open surgery for rectal cancer. N Engl J Med. 2015;373(2):194.
21. Bosshardt TL. Outcomes of ostomy procedures in patients aged 70 years and older. Arch Surg. 2003;138(10):1077–82.

18 Hepatobiliary Surgery

Giorgio Ercolani, Riccardo Turrini, Eleonora Pozzi, and Valentina Zucchini

18.1 Introduction

Malignant liver tumors, both primary and secondary, are more commonly diagnosed in people aged over 65 years and, owing to aging of the general population, the incidence is steadily growing [1]. Surgical resection remains the best chance of cure for patients, but perioperative management is often more challenging than in other types of surgery. When evaluating a patient for hepatic resection (HR), oncological factors must be balanced with the need to preserve an adequate future liver remnant to ensure postoperative function. In elderly patients, this may be particularly challenging due to reduced hepatic regenerative capacity [2]. Moreover, limited life expectancy should be taken into account when considering oncologic surgery in this population since it could limit the survival benefit of surgery [3].

HR requires complex perioperative management, even from an anesthesiologic perspective. Intraoperative strategies primarily focus on minimizing hepatic bleeding; however, in patients with reduced cardiovascular tolerance to hypotension and hypoperfusion, the traditional low central venous pressure approach may be difficult to implement. Even routine maneuvers in hepatic surgery, such as portal triad clamping (which causes reduced cardiac output due to elevation in systemic vascular resistance and mean arterial pressure) can be problematic because of aging-related impairment of compensatory reflexes, even in the absence of significant comorbidities [4].

The advancements in surgical techniques, systemic therapies and perioperative management have extended the eligibility of older people for liver resections [1].

G. Ercolani · R. Turrini (✉) · E. Pozzi · V. Zucchini
Pierantoni-Morgagni General Hospital, Department of Medical and Surgical Sciences (DIMEC), Alma Mater Studiorum University of Bologna, Bologna, Italy
e-mail: giorgio.ercolani2@unibo.it; riccardo.turrini2@studio.unibo.it; eleonora.pozzi3@studio.unibo.it; vale.zucchini94@gmail.com

P. Carcoforo, F. Catena (eds.), *Geriatric Surgery*, Updates in Surgery,
https://doi.org/10.1007/978-3-032-24281-5_18

The most common malignant liver tumors differ in their natural history and characteristics. Most hepatic resections are performed for colorectal liver metastases, which are generally associated with good overall survival (OS) [5]. Even among primary tumors, hepatocarcinoma (HCC) and cholangiocarcinoma have shown to have distinct outcomes and treatment strategies, and will therefore be discussed separately in this chapter.

18.2 Colorectal Liver Metastasis

Colorectal cancer (CRC) is the second most common cancer in Europe [6], with a rising global incidence [7, 8]. About 27% of CRC patients develop liver metastases (CRLM) within 5 years of CRC diagnosis [5]. Surgical resection remains the only potentially curative option, with a 5-year survival rate of nearly 50% [5].

Despite an overall increase in HRs worldwide [9], this trend does not extend to patients over 75, who are also less likely to undergo major resections [9, 10]. A 2018 North American study on patients with stage IV CRC [11] showed a decline in HR rates with age: patients aged 76–80 were half as likely to undergo HR compared to those aged 66–70 (odds ratio [OR] 0.50; 95% CI: 0.35–0.60; $p < 0.001$), and only 1.4% of patients >85 received surgery, compared to 7% of 66–70 years old. Referrals for surgical evaluation also decreased with age (OR 0.42 for age 81–85; $p < 0.001$), suggesting an age-related disparity in both evaluation and treatment.

Although no randomized controlled trials have defined the optimal management in elderly patients, several reviews and meta-analyses have addressed this topic. Some report lower 5-year OS in patients aged >70 or >75, but no differences in 3- and 5-year disease-free survival (DFS) or clear margin (R0) resection rates after HR [12, 13]. This suggests that the increased mortality may be driven by non-cancer-related causes, especially considering that older patients often present with more comorbidities.

Regarding short-term outcomes, van Tuil et al. [13] found no significant difference in postoperative morbidity between the <70 and > 70 age groups (27% vs. 30% respectively, $p = 0.35$), nor in hospital stay (12.6 ± 11.6 vs. 13.2 ± 10.7 days, $p = 0.19$). However, mortality was higher in older patients (4% vs. 2% respectively, $p = 0.01$). In those >75, morbidity was 32% (vs. 21% in younger patients, $p = 0.001$), and postoperative mortality was 6% (vs. 1%, $p = 0.02$) after HR.

These data are consistent with another meta-analysis [13] showing increased 30-day mortality in patients aged >70 compared to younger patients (OR 1.92; 95% CI: 1.12–3.31; $p = 0.02$), despite a similar complication rate. A French meta-analysis [14] also found no significant difference in Clavien ≥III complications between older and younger patients. Thus, the authors suggest that higher postoperative mortality may result from complications having a greater impact in elderly patients.

In recent years, increasing evidence has also emerged supporting the use of laparoscopic hepatectomy (LH) approaches in elderly patients. Indeed, a 2017 prospective multicenter cohort study [15] included 775 patients aged >70 years undergoing HR for CRLM and found no differences in postoperative complications between laparoscopic and open hepatectomies in patients aged >80 years. However, when considering the entire cohort, after propensity score matching, LH was associated with lower intraoperative blood loss, reduce use of Pringle maneuver, shorter hospital stay, and lower overall complication rates, including respiratory tract infections. Also, no differences in recurrence-free survival or OS were observed.

Another relevant issue is the optimal timing of HR for synchronous CRLM. Currently, no consensus exists, due to the lack of randomized controlled trials. In the general population, simultaneous resection has been linked to higher postoperative risk, especially with major hepatectomy [16]. A multi-society guideline [17] recommends tailoring the surgical strategy to liver disease burden and patient frailty. Some studies found increased complication rates in patients >70 undergoing simultaneous resection [18, 19], and recommended that major hepatectomies should be approached with caution in patients aged >75 owing to the increased postoperative risk [17].

However, available studies have several limitations: the age cut-offs defining "elderly" vary widely across studies (from >65 to >85). Moreover, most of the studies are retrospective, and therefore subject to selection bias, typically including only patients with better performance status.

Frailty has thus emerged as a more accurate predictor of surgical risk than chronological age alone. A recent meta-analysis including 71,102 patients [20] found frailty significantly associated with major complications (e.g., postoperative liver failure), mortality, and readmission. Although correlated with age, frailty was also independently associated with lower albumin levels, indicating poor nutritional status.

Furthermore, a prospective study of 1826 patients [21] confirmed that frailty predicted worse postoperative outcomes regardless of age. Frail patients, both younger and older, had more complications, longer hospital stays, and higher mortality compared to non-frail patients. These findings suggest that frailty, rather than chronological age alone, is a more accurate predictor of postoperative risk in patients undergoing HR.

18.3 Hepatocellular Carcinoma

Hepatocellular carcinoma (HCC) is the most common primary liver cancer worldwide, representing 75–85% of cases, and the second leading cause of cancer-related mortality [22, 23]. Chronic viral hepatitis remains the major risk factor (HBV in Asia-Pacific and Africa, HCV in Western countries). However, in high-income regions, the rising prevalence of metabolic factors (obesity, diabetes, and nonalcoholic fatty liver disease) is becoming increasingly relevant [23]. These conditions predispose to HCC over time, with the highest age-specific rates observed in individuals aged ≥70 years, especially in Western countries where the overall incidence is lower [24].

HCC management is multimodal and requires multidisciplinary evaluation, as it is intrinsically linked to liver function; more than 80–90% of cases occur in cirrhotic livers [25]. The TNM staging system is limited, as it disregards liver function and overall patient's health status [26]. Alternative prognostic classifications have been proposed, the most widely used in Europe being the Barcelona-Clinic Liver Cancer (BCLC) classification [27]. This system incorporates performance status for prognosis and treatment allocation; although older patients often present with worse performance status, chronological age alone is not considered as a prognostic factor.

Treatment options include locoregional therapies, such as liver transplantation (LT), surgical resection, ablation, transarterial chemoembolization (TACE), or radioembolization (TARE), and several systemic therapies. International hepato-pancreato-biliary (HPB) guidelines propose algorithms based on tumor burden, liver function, and patient condition, often integrating prognostic scores to guide multidisciplinary decisions [3, 28, 29]. Only resection, ablation, and LT are potentially curative [30]. In non-cirrhotic livers with preserved function, surgical resection or ablation (when surgery is unfeasible) are preferred [3]. For cirrhotic livers, LT offers definitive treatment of both cancer and cirrhosis but carries drawbacks: lifestyle changes, immunosuppression therapies and risk of waitlist dropout, due to disease progression or, particularly in older patients, clinical deterioration [3].

Thirty years ago, LT was not even considered for patients aged >60 years. Advances in surgical techniques and perioperative care have extended eligibility, with no absolute upper age limit. In 2016, more than 30% of European LT recipients were >60 years old, with 10-year survival rates of 40% among septuagenarians [31]. Similar U.S. data show 23% of recipients in 2020 were >65, of whom 30% had HCC [32]. Despite feasibility, given organ scarcity, prioritization often favors younger recipients, even though older patients can achieve acceptable long-term survival, in some countries patients >65 are not eligible for LT [28].

When feasible, resection remains the preferred treatment in older patients, depending on tumor stage, site, and hepatic function. A recent meta-analysis, including 56 studies from Asia and Europe, suggests comparable DFS and cancer-specific mortality rates between elderly and younger cohorts after R0 resection [33]. Evidence on short-term outcomes is conflicting: some meta-analysis report higher rates of minor complications but no difference in major events or post-hepatectomy liver failure, while others indicate increased morbidity and mortality, particularly in patients aged >80 years [33, 34]. However, most studies are retrospective and limited by inadequate adjustment for comorbidities. What appears to be clear instead is that minimally invasive approaches (laparoscopic or robotic) are consistently associated with fewer complications, reduced post-hepatectomy liver failure, and shorter hospitalization, most of the times with greater benefit in the elderly, obtaining comparable oncological outcomes [35, 36].

Given these data, the most recent European guidelines state that age alone should not contraindicate surgical resection. Instead, comorbidities and frailty represent more reliable prognostic tools. Years of life lost is also recommended as an evaluation parameter instead of patient's age [3]. In elderly patients with high comorbidity burden or limited life expectancy, thermal ablation should be considered, even with favorable liver function or future liver remnant after resection, owing to lower perioperative morbidity and mortality [37].

18.4 Intrahepatic Cholangiocarcinoma

Intrahepatic cholangiocarcinoma is the second most common primary liver cancer after HCC, with over 75% of cases diagnosed at ≥65 years. Prognosis is poor due to late diagnosis, aggressiveness, and resistance to therapy, with 5-year survival <10% [38].

Older age is a known risk factor. Chronic biliary inflammation is the main pathogenic mechanism, though no risk factor is identified in up to 70% of cases [38]. Surgical resection with negative margins remains the only curative treatment, typically through segmentectomy or extended hemihepatectomy. Only 12–40% of cases are resectable at diagnosis, and recurrence is common, with 5-year OS between 25% and 40% [39]. An adequate remanant liver volume is crucial and must be ≥25–30% in healthy livers and >40% in fibrotic/steatotic ones, conditions more frequently found in the elderly. Data from large cohorts [40, 41] show lower treatment intensity with age: patients aged ≥75 are less likely to receive surgery or systemic therapy. In contrast, those aged 65–74 more often undergo chemotherapy or surgery ± chemotherapy. Surgery appears to provide the most consistent survival benefit, whereas the addition of chemotherapy does not clearly improve prognosis.

Available evidence [40, 41] suggests tumor stage and nodal status are stronger survival predictors than age. Octogenarians tend to undergo less extensive resections but achieve comparable R0 and lymphadenectomy rates. Despite longer intensive care unit stays and higher perioperative risk, outcomes in selected elderly patients match younger cohorts.Minimally invasive surgery for lesions <5 cm in favorable locations can reduce morbidity without compromising oncologic results. Robotic surgery may increase precision, but data in older patients are limited [42].

For frail patients unfit for resection, local ablation or stereotactic radiotherapy may offer disease control; intra-arterial therapies remain investigational.

18.5 Perihilar Cholangiocarcinoma

Perihilar cholangiocarcinoma, or Klatskin tumor, originates at the biliary confluence and accounts for 50–60% of cholangiocarcinomas, peaking between 60 and 80 years [43].

It is usually diagnosed late, following jaundice onset. Advanced stages respond poorly to chemotherapy, and surgery is the only curative option.

The Bismuth-Corlette classification (I–IV) remains standard.

High bilirubin raises surgical risk. Preoperative hyperbilirubinemia markedly increases postoperative risk: ESMO (European Society for Medical Oncology) [39] indicates drainage when bilirubin >250 μmol/L (~14.6 mg/dL), while ESGE (European Society of Gastrointestinal Endoscopy) [44] and ASGE (American Society for Gastrointestinal Endoscopy) [45] prefer a case-by-case assessment.

Absolute indications include cholangitis, sepsis, intractable pruritus, severe jaundice (>15 mg/dL), and candidates for neoadjuvant therapy or procedures such as portal vein embolization. Endoscopic retrograde cholangiopancreatography is preferred for Bismuth I–II, whereas percutaneous drainage is recommended for types III–IV to decompress both lobes. In elderly patients with obstruction, endoscopic approaches are favored for their lower complication rate, though percutaneous transhepatic biliary drainage may be required if endoscopy fails.

Curative surgery involves bile duct resection, major hepatectomy, and hepatoduodenal lymphadenectomy. Extended right hepatectomy is the most common approach, facilitated by the longer left hepatic duct and often preceded by right portal vein embolization [39].

Liver failure is the leading cause of postoperative death, often linked to extended resections in the setting of cholestasis or cholangitis. Risk factors include age, hypoalbuminemia, cholangitis, hyperbilirubinemia, transfusions, vascular resections, and incomplete biliary drainage.

Short-term mortality rises with age, especially in octogenarians, who show a higher risk of death at 30 and 90 days compared with younger cohorts [46]. However, elderly patients more often present with early-stage disease (Bismuth I–II, American Joint Committee on Cancer [AJCC] I–III), enabling less aggressive surgery with R0 rates and long-term outcomes comparable when resection is performed [46, 47].

Despite higher early risk, surgery remains the only route to long-term survival in non-metastatic perihilar cholangiocarcinoma, as survival beyond 3 years without resection is rare. Outcomes in fit elderly patients mirror younger cohorts, though selection bias likely plays a role. With rising life expectancy, age alone should not exclude patients from surgery, tumor biology and stage remain the main prognostic factors.

18.6 Gallbladder Cancer

Gallbladder cancer (GBC) is a rare malignancy, ranking sixth among gastrointestinal malignancies [48]. Incidental GBC, diagnosed after cholecystectomy, occurs in 0.3–1.5% of cases, rising to 9% in patients ≥80 years [49]. Median age at diagnosis is 70, with higher risk in women [50].

Prognosis remains poor, with 5-year survival rates of 67% for localized, 29% for regional, and 4% for metastatic disease, worsening with age [51].

For stages beyond T1a, re-resection is advised when feasible, involving partial hepatectomy of segments IVb-V and hepatoduodenal lymphadenectomy [39]. Advanced T stage is not a contraindication for fundic tumors, but infundibular lesions may require multivisceral resections with high morbidity. Some evidence [49] supports surgical benefit in selected patients aged 70–84, but outcomes worsen in those ≥85 due to frailty and higher risk. Recurrence is common (~80% within 3 years), warranting evaluation of adjuvant therapy. Trials in elderly patients are limited. An analysis of data from the Surveillance, Epidemiology, and End Results SEER database [49] showed no OS benefit from adjuvant chemotherapy in those ≥65, whereas another study [52] found improved survival in node-positive, advanced-stage patients (T3/T4).

The BILCAP trial [53] suggested a benefit from capecitabine in per-protocol analyses, and this is now recommended in several guidelines for biliary tract cancers, including GBC.

18.7 Conclusions

Based on the most recent evidence, both minor and major hepatic resections are feasible in elderly patients. Advances in surgical techniques –particularly minimally invasive approaches—together with improvements in perioperative management have yielded significant benefits in survival and short-term outcomes, even within this population. A multiparametric assessment of frailty appears to provide a more reliable measure than chronological age when evaluating candidates for hepatic resection.

References

1. Petrowsky H, Clavien PA. Should we deny surgery for malignant hepato-pancreatico-biliary tumors to elderly patients? World J Surg. 2005;29(9):1093–100.
2. Sturesson C, Nilsson J, Eriksson S, et al. Limiting factors for liver regeneration after a major hepatic resection for colorectal cancer metastases. HPB (Oxford). 2013;15:646–52.
3. European Association for the Study of the Liver. EASL Clinical Practice Guidelines on the management of hepatocellular carcinoma. J Hepatol. 2025;82:315–74.
4. Wallace H, Miller T, Angus W, Stott M. Intra-operative anaesthetic management of older patients undergoing liver surgery. Eur J Surg Oncol. 2021;47(3 Pt A):545–50.
5. Engstrand J, Nilsson H, Strömberg C, et al. Colorectal cancer liver metastases – a population-based study on incidence, management and survival. BMC Cancer. 2018;18(1):78.
6. Dyba T, Randi G, Bray F, et al. The European cancer burden in 2020: incidence and mortality estimates for 40 countries and 25 major cancers. Eur J Cancer. 2021;157:308–47.
7. Morgan E, Arnold M, Gini A, et al. Global burden of colorectal cancer in 2020 and 2040: incidence and mortality estimates from GLOBOCAN. Gut. 2023;72(2):338–44.
8. Vuik FE, Nieuwenburg SA, Bardou M, et al. Increasing incidence of colorectal cancer in young adults in Europe over the last 25 years. Gut. 2019;68(10):1820–6.
9. Booth CM, Nanji S, Wei X, Mackillop WJ. Management and outcome of colorectal cancer liver metastases in elderly patients: a population-based study. JAMA Oncol. 2015;1(8):1111–9.
10. Tzeng CWD, Cooper AB, Vauthey JN, et al. Predictors of morbidity and mortality after hepatectomy in elderly patients: analysis of 7621 NSQIP patients. HPB (Oxford). 2014;16(5):459–68.
11. Neuwirth MG, Epstein AJ, Karakousis GC, et al. Disparities in resection of hepatic metastases in colon cancer. J Gastrointest Oncol. 2018;9(1):126–34.
12. Xie M, Zhu J, He X, et al. Liver metastasis from colorectal cancer in the elderly: is surgery justified? Dig Dis Sci. 2015;60(12):3525–35.
13. van Tuil T, Dhaif AA, te Riele WW, et al. Systematic review and meta-analysis of liver resection for colorectal metastases in elderly patients. Dig Surg. 2019;36(2):111–23.
14. de'Angelis N, Baldini C, Brustia R, et al. Surgical and regional treatments for colorectal cancer metastases in older patients: a systematic review and meta-analysis. PLoS One. 2020;15(4):e0230914.

15. Martínez-Cecilia D, Cipriani F, Shelat V, et al. Laparoscopic versus open liver resection for colorectal metastases in elderly and octogenarian patients: a multicenter propensity score based analysis of short- and long-term outcomes. Ann Surg. 2017;265(6):1192–200.
16. Radomski SN, Chen SY, Stem M, et al. Simultaneous resection of colorectal cancer and synchronous colorectal liver metastases: a risk stratified analysis of the NSQIP database. J Surg Oncol. 2023;128(7):1095–105.
17. Podda M, Sylla P, Baiocchi G, et al. Multidisciplinary management of elderly patients with rectal cancer: recommendations from the SICG (Italian Society of Geriatric Surgery), SIFIPAC (Italian Society of Surgical Pathophysiology), SICE (Italian Society of Endoscopic Surgery and new technologies), and the WSES (World Society of Emergency Surgery) international consensus project. World J Emerg Surg. 2021;16(1):35.
18. Yin Z, Liu C, Chen Y, et al. Timing of hepatectomy in resectable synchronous colorectal liver metastases (SCRLM): simultaneous or delayed? Hepatology. 2013;57(6):2346–57.
19. Chen Q, Zhang Y, Deng Y, et al. Outcomes of simultaneous resection for elderly patients with colorectal liver metastasis: a propensity score matching analysis. Cancer Med. 2022;11(24):4913–26.
20. Lunca S, Morarasu S, Rouet K, et al. Frailty increases morbidity and mortality in patients undergoing oncological liver resections: a systematic review and meta-analysis. Ann Surg Oncol. 2024;31(10):6514–25.
21. Lv YJ, Xu GX, Lan JR. Impact of frailty on postoperative outcomes after hepatectomy: a systematic review and meta-analysis. World J Gastrointest Surg. 2024;16(7):2319–28.
22. Global Burden of Disease 2019 Cancer Collaboration, Kocarnik JM, Compton K, et al. Cancer incidence, mortality, years of life lost, years lived with disability, and disability-adjusted life years for 29 cancer groups from 2010 to 2019: a systematic analysis for the Global Burden of Disease Study 2019. JAMA Oncol. 2022;8(3):420–44.
23. Bray F, Laversanne M, Sung H, et al. Global cancer statistics 2022: GLOBOCAN estimates of incidence and mortality worldwide for 36 cancers in 185 countries. CA Cancer J Clin. 2024;74(3):229–63.
24. El-Serag HB, Rudolph KL. Hepatocellular carcinoma: epidemiology and molecular carcinogenesis. Gastroenterology. 2007;132(7):2557–76.
25. Lee DH, Lee JM. Primary malignant tumours in the non-cirrhotic liver. Eur J Radiol. 2017;95:349–61.
26. Amin MB, Greene FL, Edge SB, et al. The eighth edition AJCC Cancer Staging Manual: continuing to build a bridge from a population-based to a more "personalized" approach to cancer staging. CA Cancer J Clin. 2017;67(2):93–9.
27. Reig M, Forner A, Rimola J, et al. BCLC strategy for prognosis prediction and treatment recommendation: the 2022 update. J Hepatol. 2022;76(3):681–93.
28. Hasegawa K, Takemura N, Yamashita T, et al. Clinical Practice Guidelines for hepatocellular carcinoma: the Japan Society of Hepatology 2021 version (5th JSH-HCC Guidelines). Hepatol Res. 2023;53(5):383–90.
29. Singal AG, Llovet JM, Yarchoan M, et al. AASLD Practice Guidance on prevention, diagnosis, and treatment of hepatocellular carcinoma. Hepatology. 2023;78(6):1922–65.
30. Cucchetti A, Elshaarawy O, Han G, et al. 'Potentially curative therapies' for hepatocellular carcinoma: how many patients can actually be cured? Br J Cancer. 2023;128(9):1665–71.
31. Adam R, Karam V, Cailliez V, et al. 2018 Annual report of the European Liver Transplant Registry (ELTR) – 50-year evolution of liver transplantation. Transpl Int. 2018;31(12):1293–317.
32. Stepanova M, Kabbara K, Mohess D, et al. Nonalcoholic steatohepatitis is the most common indication for liver transplantation among the elderly: data from the United States Scientific Registry of Transplant Recipients. Hepatol Commun. 2022;6(7):1506–15.
33. Lee JS, Park DA, Ryoo S, et al. Efficacy and safety of surgical resection in elderly patients with hepatocellular carcinoma: a systematic review and meta-analysis. Gut Liver. 2024;18(4):695–708.

34. Garcia EM, Nerurkar SN, Tan EX, et al. Characteristics and outcomes of elderly hepatocellular carcinoma patients following surgical resection: systematic review and meta-analysis. Dig Dis. 2025;43(2):206–14.
35. Yoo JJ, Park DA, Ryoo S, et al. Comparing laparoscopic and open resection in elderly hepatocellular carcinoma: a systematic review and meta-analysis. J Gastrointest Oncol. 2024;15(3):1153–64.
36. Chen K, Pan Y, Maher H, et al. Laparoscopic hepatectomy for elderly patients: major findings based on a systematic review and meta-analysis. Medicine (Baltimore). 2018;97(30):e11703.
37. Yoo JJ, Koo S, Choi GH, et al. Radiofrequency ablation versus surgical resection in elderly hepatocellular carcinoma: a systematic review and meta-analysis. Curr Oncol. 2024;31(1):324–34.
38. European Association for the Study of the Liver. EASL-ILCA Clinical Practice Guidelines on the management of intrahepatic cholangiocarcinoma. J Hepatol. 2023;79(1):181–208.
39. Vogel A, Bridgewater J, Edeline J, et al. Biliary tract cancer: ESMO Clinical Practice Guideline for diagnosis, treatment and follow-up. Ann Oncol. 2023;34(2):127–40.
40. Zhu H, Ji K, Wu W, et al. Describing treatment patterns for elderly patients with intrahepatic cholangiocarcinoma and predicting prognosis by a validated model: a population-based study. J Cancer. 2021;12(11):3114–25.
41. Bangolo A, Nagesh VK, Tran HHV, et al. Age and tumor stage interplay in intrahepatic cholangiocarcinoma: prognostic factors, mortality trends, and therapeutic implications from a SEER-based analysis. Diseases. 2025;13(2):31.
42. Riffat F, Chu F, Morris DL. Liver resection in octogenarians. HPB (Oxford). 2006;8(3):206–10.
43. Sharma P, Yadav S. Demographics, tumor characteristics, treatment, and survival of patients with Klatskin tumors. Ann Gastroenterol. 2018;31(2):231–6.
44. Dumonceau JM, Tringali A, Blero D, et al. Biliary stenting: indications, choice of stents and results: European Society of Gastrointestinal Endoscopy (ESGE) clinical guideline. Endoscopy. 2012;44(3):277–98.
45. ASGE Standards of Practice Committee, Pawa S, Marya NB, et al. American society for Gastrointestinal Endoscopy guideline on the role of therapeutic EUS in the management of biliary tract disorders: summary and recommendations. Gastrointest Endosc. 2024;100(6):967–79.
46. Ripamonti L, De Carlis R, Lauterio A, et al. Major hepatectomy for perihilar cholangiocarcinoma in elderly patients: is it reasonable? Updat Surg. 2022;74(1):203–11.
47. Yu M, Lu L, Wu R. Perihilar cholangiocarcinoma resection: is it beneficial for survival in elderly patients? Gastroenterol Hepatol. 2024;47(7):691–701.
48. Halaseh SA, Halaseh S, Shakman R. A review of the etiology and epidemiology of gallbladder cancer: what you need to know. Cureus. 2022;14(8):e28260.
49. Xu X, Wang J, Duan Q. Effects of surgery on survival of elderly patients with gallbladder cancer: a propensity score matching analysis of the SEER database. Front Oncol. 2023;13:1083618.
50. Coburn NG, Cleary SP, Tan JCC, Law CHL. Surgery for gallbladder cancer: a population-based analysis. J Am Coll Surg. 2008;207(3):371–82.
51. Guragain A, Inban P, Vaz C, et al. Survival of primary gallbladder cancer in the United States: SEER database analysis from 2000-2020. J Clin Oncol. 2024;42(16 Suppl):e16210.
52. de Savornin Lohman E, Belkouz A, Nuliyalu U, et al. Adjuvant treatment for the elderly patient with resected gallbladder cancer: a SEER-Medicare analysis. J Gastrointest Oncol. 2022;13(6):3227239.
53. Rizzo A, Brandi G. BILCAP trial and adjuvant capecitabine in resectable biliary tract cancer: reflections on a standard of care. Expert Rev Gastroenterol Hepatol. 2021;15(5):483–5.

Abdominal Wall Surgery

19

Gagik Beglaryan, Piero Giovanni Bruni, Marta Cavalli, Livia Manfredini, Niccolò Grappolini, and Giampiero Campanelli

19.1 Introduction

Abdominal wall pathology in geriatric patients represents a special challenge to be treated with specialized management and customized surgical approaches [1, 2]. As the global population ages, surgeons are confronted with an increasing volume of elderly patients with complex abdominal wall defects, hernias, and reconstruction needs. Physiological changes of aging, including decreased tissue elasticity, impaired wound healing, muscle mass, and increased comorbidities, significantly influence surgical planning and outcomes in the elderly [3].

Abdominal wall surgery represents a broad spectrum of procedures, from the simple hernia repair to complex reconstructions of the many components of the abdominal wall [4]. In elderly patients, these procedures must be carefully balanced against the need for definitive treatment and the risks of old age [5]. The incidence of abdominal wall hernias increases with age, with inguinal hernias in approximately 13% of men over 65 years and incisional hernias more common after abdominal surgery in this group [6].

Improved surgical technique, anesthetic practice, and perioperative care that have followed recent advances have provided a greater scope for the treatment of the elderly with abdominal wall disease [7, 8].

Nonetheless, in the majority of cases, successful outcomes require diligent preoperative assessment, proper selection of surgical techniques, and appropriate postoperative care tailored to the unique features of the elderly patient.

G. Beglaryan · P. G. Bruni · M. Cavalli · L. Manfredini · N. Grappolini · G. Campanelli (✉)
IRCCS Ospedale Galeazzi – Sant'Ambrogio (Hernia Center Milano), University of Insubria, Milan, Italy
e-mail: giampiero.campanelli@grupposandonato.it

P. Carcoforo, F. Catena (eds.), *Geriatric Surgery*, Updates in Surgery, https://doi.org/10.1007/978-3-032-24281-5_19

19.2 Epidemiology and Risk Factors

19.2.1 Prevalence of Abdominal Wall Hernias in the Elderly

The incidence of abdominal wall hernias increases markedly with increasing age, and consequently hernia repair is among the most common surgical procedures in elderly patients [1, 6]. Inguinal hernias occur particularly in elderly men, with a lifetime risk of almost 27% and a prevalence of almost 13% among men over the age of 65 years [1, 6]. The risk continues to increase with advancing age, though peak incidence rates are in men over the age of 75 years.

Incisional hernias are yet another important category of abdominal wall pathology in the elderly [5]. Incisional hernia after abdominal surgery is 10–20% in the general population. However, the prevalence is extremely high in the elderly owing to factors such as defective wound healing, increased comorbidities, and the higher probability of prior abdominal surgery [9]. The rate of incisional hernia is very high after emergency procedures, which are more common among the elderly [10].

Ventral hernias, including epigastric and umbilical hernias, also show increased incidence with advancing age [4]. Age-related degradation of the linea alba and the other fascial components predisposes the geriatric patient to the development of these hernias that may be complicated defects requiring complicated reconstruction techniques [11].

19.2.2 Risk Factors Specific to the Elderly Population

Certain risk factors for abdominal wall hernia and complications are particularly applicable to elderly groups [1, 12]. Age alone is an independent risk factor beyond other influences, and the relative risk of hernia increases by approximately 1.5–2 fold with each decade above the age of 50 years [6]. Chronic diseases, such as chronic obstructive pulmonary disease (COPD) with chronic cough and increased intra-abdominal pressure, significantly increase the risk of hernia [13].

Obesity, although less common in the elderly, remains a high risk factor if it is present [12], whereas sarcopenia and muscle loss compromise the intrinsic supporting structures of the abdominal wall [12].

Chronic medical conditions such as diabetes mellitus, cardiovascular disease, and chronic kidney disease not only predispose to hernia development but also complicate surgical management and postoperative recovery [1, 14].

19.3 Preoperative Evaluation and Optimization

19.3.1 Cardiac and Pulmonary Evaluation

Cardiovascular evaluation of the elderly patient presenting for abdominal wall surgery must follow the established principles of perioperative cardiac risk evaluation [1].

The American College of Cardiology/American Heart Association guidelines provide a strategy for cardiac risk assessment based on the nature of the surgery, patient characteristics of risk, and functional status. Most hernia operations are low-risk procedures; however, more complex abdominal wall reconstructions would qualify as intermediate-risk procedures [15, 16].

Pulmonary function tests are indicated in the elderly since pulmonary complications are one of the most common perioperative complications in this population [13]. Preoperative pulmonary function testing may be necessary in those with severe respiratory symptoms or a history of lung disease. Tests should include evaluation for chronic obstructive pulmonary disease, asthma, and other processes that may affect perioperative management.

Preoperative optimization of both pulmonary and cardiac status can significantly improve outcome [1, 13]. This may include optimization of medication, treatment of heart failure, treatment of COPD with bronchodilators, and offering smoking cessation counseling. The operation may be delayed to allow optimization of status, particularly in non-emergency surgery.

19.3.2 Anesthetic Considerations

When choosing the type of anesthesia in the older patient for repair of the abdominal wall we must consider both the physiological alterations of old age and the patient's comorbidities [1, 17]. Local anesthesia with sedation may be appropriate for simple repairs in order to minimize the overall impact of anesthesia. Spinal or epidural anesthesia may provide good operating conditions without the risk of respiratory depression that can be caused of the general anesthesia [7].

General anesthesia may be necessary in cases of complex surgery or patient-related factors that are a contraindication to the use of regional techniques [1]. More recently developed anesthetic agents with rapid onset and recovery can prevent the risks of prolonged sedation and cognitive impairment in the elderly. The anesthetic technique has to be individualized based on the patient's past history, functional status, and nature of planned surgery [13].

19.4 Surgical Techniques and Considerations

19.4.1 Principles of Hernia Repair in the Elderly

The fundamental principles of hernia repair in the elderly patient are the same as in young adults, but need to be modified to accommodate physiological decline with increasing age and a higher burden of comorbid illness [2]. The general goals remain the same: close the defect, restore abdominal wall integrity, and prevent recurrence with the goal to decrease morbidity and mortality. However, the approach to achieving these goals must be modified in line with the unique needs and limitations of the geriatric patient population.

The term "physiological hernia repair" has become more popular in older patients, in whom one needs to tailor the surgical technique according to the life expectancy and physiological reserve of the patient [3]. This can involve accepting a higher recurrence rate for decreased morbidity and mortality, especially in life-limited or comorbid patients.

Tension-free techniques are now the gold standard for most hernia repairs and are particularly important in the elderly, where tissue quality may be compromised [7]. Mesh reinforcement allows repair to be accomplished without putting undue tension on compromised tissues, minimizing the risk of recurrence and maximizing patient comfort throughout the healing process.

19.4.2 Inguinal Hernia Repair with Local Anesthesia

Inguinal hernia repair under local anesthesia can be considered as the best approach of treatment in the elderly patient. It is associated with numerous advantages such as reduced systemic complications, early mobilization, and improved patient satisfaction. Hernia repair through the use of local anesthetic mesh is safe and effective in elderly patients and is an extremely useful approach in the elderly [17].

19.4.3 Patient Selection and Contraindications

Local anesthesia is particularly ideal for elderly patients with several comorbidities who will not be able to tolerate general or regional anesthesia. Some of the ideal candidates are cardiac or pulmonary patients, those receiving anticoagulation therapy, or those who have had previous difficult intubation or anesthetic complications.

Relative contraindications include patient anxiety or uncooperation, recurrent hernias with extensive scarring, large scrotal hernias requiring extensive dissection, and perhaps hernias with suspected bowel involvement. Operative skills are also necessary, as in challenging cases general anesthesia may be necessary.

19.4.4 Outcomes and Advantages

Studies report favorable outcomes of inguinal hernia repair under local anesthesia in the elderly. Recurrence rates are comparable to those with general anesthesia, at 1–3% at 5-year follow-up. There are several added advantages of the technique in the elderly, including decreased postoperative vomiting and nausea, quick recovery of bowel function, reduced risk of urinary retention, and earlier mobilization.

The ability to assess the repair intraoperatively, by asking the patient to cough or perform Valsalva maneuvers, provides the surgeon with an immediate measure of whether or not the repair is sufficient. Such immediate feedback allows the surgeon to identify areas of weakness that require reinforcement.

19.4.5 Ventral Incisional Hernia Repair

Ventral incisional hernias are a significant challenge in elderly patients, with incidence rates of 10–20% following abdominal surgery, increasing exponentially with age due to impaired wound healing and the presence of various comorbid diseases [5]. Management of such complicated defects requires refined balancing of patient variables, defect size and characteristics, and available surgical options.

19.4.6 Preoperative Planning and Evaluation

Computed tomography scan gives precise information regarding defect size, defect site, and number of defects. The width of the rectus muscle and the extent of lateral retraction need to be measured, as these determine the potential for fascial closure and the requirement for component separation techniques [4].

The retromuscular (sublay) technique is also gaining wider acceptance as the operation of choice in open ventral hernia repair in elderly patients. The procedure provides optimal mesh coverage with well-vascularized tissue and maintains the mesh in an extraperitoneal position, reducing adhesions and bowel complications [12].

Component separation techniques can be employed in large defects where closure of both anterior and/or posterior compartments is not possible.

19.4.7 Laparoscopic Ventral Hernia Repair

Laparoscopic intraperitoneal onlay mesh ventral hernia repair offers significant benefits in elderly patients, such as less postoperative pain, shorter hospitalization, and lower wound complication rates [15]. It is especially beneficial for elderly patients with several comorbid diseases who are likely to benefit from the decreased physiological stress of minimally invasive procedures.

19.4.8 Mesh Selection for Ventral Hernia Repair

Lightweight polypropylene meshes with large pore size have been the most preferred for many applications due to the fact that they induce less foreign body reaction and greater patient comfort. These meshes provide greater tissue ingrowth while the meshes continue to supply sufficient strength for hernia repair. The reduced inflammatory reaction can prove particularly beneficial in older patients who have impaired healing.

Biologic or biosynthetic meshes derived from animal or human tissue offer an advantage in infected fields or for high-risk patients. These are, however, more costly and possibly the risk of recurrence is higher [14]. In older patients with limited life expectancy, the higher rate of recurrence can be accepted at the cost of reduced complications.

Composite meshes with different surfaces for visceral and parietal contact have been developed for intraperitoneal placement. The meshes consist of a non-adherent surface facing the bowel and an ingrowth surface facing the abdominal wall. Although these meshes reduce the formation of adhesions, they are at risk of being associated with high rates of seroma in older patients.

19.4.9 Minimally Invasive Techniques

Minimally invasive surgical techniques such as laparoscopic and robotic techniques have revolutionized hernia repair and are particularly useful in the elderly population [18]. These techniques are associated with smaller wounds, decreased postoperative pain, reduced hospital stay, and faster return to normal activities. There is evidence to believe that minimally invasive surgery improves recovery and decreases postoperative morbidity in the elderly and is therefore a desirable option in the elderly.

Laparoscopic techniques of inguinal hernia repair, i.e., totally extraperitoneal (TEP) and transabdominal preperitoneal (TAPP) repairs, have the advantages of good visualization of anatomy and enable contralateral hernia detection and repair [7]. These are particularly useful in recurrent, bilateral or ventral hernias. Laparoscopic procedures have a steep learning curve, but, in experienced hands, excellent results can be obtained in the elderly.

19.4.10 Outcomes and Prognosis

Recurrence rates for hernioplasty in elderly patients are generally comparable to those in younger patients if contemporary techniques are utilized [7, 19]. Recurrence rate in tension-free inguinal hernioplasty is generally less than 5% at 5 years in all ages [2]. Recurrence rates may be greater, however, in complicated ventral hernia repair, particularly in those who have more than a single risk factor [4, 16].

Chronic postoperative pain following hernia repair is a risk in all patients but can be particularly problematic in elderly patients [20]. Although chronic pain is rare with modern techniques, in elderly patients it can become progressively more challenging to treat due to comorbidities and medication sensitivities [1, 21].

19.5 Special Considerations

Emergency hernia surgery in the elderly presents unique issues and much greater risks than elective repair [10]. Incarceration, strangulation of hernias, obstruction, and complications of previous repairs are the most common emergency presentations [1]. Their treatment includes urgent assessment, resuscitation, and operation with appropriate consideration for the patient's overall status and prognosis [13].

Diagnosis of acute abdominal wall pathologies in the older adult may be challenged by atypical presentation and decreased pain sensation [1]. Older adults may not show symptoms and signs of typical bowel obstruction or strangulation and, as a result, have delayed diagnosis and intervention [10]. A high degree of suspicion and liberal use of imaging studies should be used for diagnosis [12].

Preoperative assessment of the elderly patient for emergency surgery must be streamlined but also cover the most critical determinants of outcome [1, 13]. The patient's cardiovascular and pulmonary status, fluid and electrolyte status, and sepsis or other such life-threatening states must be assessed [22]. There is not always an optimum time, but minor steps such as fluid replacement and correction of electrolyte imbalance must be carried out when there is time [1].

The surgical strategy for urgent operation in the geriatric patient must be directed toward a life-saving procedure with as little operative trauma as possible [10]. Simple, noncomplex measures may be employed rather than complicated reconstructions at the expense of increased recurrence risk [1]. Prosthetic material in the presence of contamination must be used with extreme caution, and biologic meshes can be the material of choice in some cases [23, 24].

Perioperative care in elderly patients who present with emergency surgery must be closely monitored and can involve intensive care unit admission [13]. Complications are much more dangerous during emergencies, and they must be diagnosed as early as possible and treated urgently for a good outcome [1].

19.6 Future Directions and Research

19.6.1 New Techniques and Technologies

Abdominal wall surgery is also progressing with new techniques and technology that may be particularly beneficial in the elderly [7, 8]. Perioperative care, technique, and materials are all improving and are expanding the scope of treatment for the elderly patient, with a potential reduction in surgery-related risks [18].

Robotic surgery is probably one of the most significant advancements in abdominal wall surgery in recent years [8]. The improved visualization and precision of robotic systems can be particularly useful in elderly patients with complex anatomy or a history of previous surgery [18].

19.6.2 Precision Medicine Approaches

Machine learning and artificial intelligence approaches are being formulated to predict outcomes and individualize therapy decisions [22]. Such a device would be particularly useful in elderly patients, where the degree of comorbidities and an appreciation of the balance of benefits and risks create difficulty in treatment decisions [1, 12].

Individualized mesh selection based on patient parameters and defect parameters is an active area of research [20, 23]. Optimal mesh type selection or patient-specific meshes based on individual patient parameters can optimize outcomes and reduce complications [21].

References

1. Perez AJ, Campbell S. Inguinal hernia repair in older persons. J Am Med Dir Assoc. 2022;23(4):563–7.
2. Simons MP, Aufenacker T, Bay-Nielsen M, et al. European Hernia Society guidelines on the treatment of inguinal hernia in adult patients. Hernia. 2009;13(4):343–403.
3. Fitzgibbons RJ Jr, Giobbie-Hurder A, Gibbs JO, et al. Watchful waiting vs repair of inguinal hernia in minimally symptomatic men: a randomized clinical trial. JAMA. 2006;295(3):285–92.
4. Liang MK, Holihan JL, Itani K, et al. Ventral hernia management: expert consensus guided by systematic review. Ann Surg. 2017;265(1):80–9.
5. Poulose BK, Shelton J, Phillips S, et al. Epidemiology and cost of ventral hernia repair: making the case for hernia research. Hernia. 2012;16(2):179–83.
6. Choi JJ, Palaniappa NC, Dallas KB, et al. Use of mesh during ventral hernia repair in clean-contaminated and contaminated cases: outcomes of 33,832 cases. Ann Surg. 2012;255(1):176–80.
7. Bittner R, Arregui ME, Bisgaard T, et al. Guidelines for laparoscopic (TAPP) and endoscopic (TEP) treatment of inguinal hernia. [International Endohernia Society (IEHS)]. Surg Endosc. 2011;25(9):2773–843.
8. Krpata DM, Petro CC, Prabhu AS, et al. Effect of hernia mesh weights on postoperative patient-related and clinical outcomes after open ventral hernia repair: a randomized clinical trial. JAMA Surg. 2021;156(12):1085–92.
9. Goh SSN, Sanghvi KA, Koura AN, et al. Elective incisional hernia repair: lower risk of postoperative wound infection with laparoscopic versus open repair. Singapore Med J. 2023;64(2):105–8.
10. Bedi AP, Bhatti T, Amin A, Zuberi J. Laparoscopic incisional and ventral hernia repair. J Minim Access Surg. 2007;3(3):83–90.
11. Martins MR, Santos-Sousa H, do Vale MA, et al. Comparison between the open and the laparoscopic approach in the primary ventral hernia repair: a systematic review and meta-analysis. Langenbecks Arch Surg. 2024;409(1):52.
12. Holihan JL, Alawadi Z, Martindale RG, et al. Adverse events after ventral hernia repair: the vicious cycle of complications. J Am Coll Surg. 2015;221(2):478–85.
13. Muysoms FE, Miserez M, Berrevoet F, et al. Classification of primary and incisional abdominal wall hernias. Hernia. 2009;13(4):407–14.
14. Rosen MJ, Krpata DM, Ermlich B, Blatnik JA. A 5-year clinical experience with single-staged repairs of infected and contaminated abdominal wall defects utilizing biologic mesh. Ann Surg. 2013;257(6):991–6.
15. Itani KM, Hur K, Kim LT, et al. Comparison of laparoscopic and open repair with mesh for the treatment of ventral incisional hernia: a randomized trial. Arch Surg. 2010;145(4):322–8.
16. Tastaldi L, Blatnik JA, Krpata DM, et al. Posterior component separation with transversus abdominis release (TAR) for repair of complex incisional hernias after orthotopic liver transplantation. Hernia. 2019;23(2):363–73.
17. Rosenberg J, Bisgaard T, Kehlet H, et al. Danish Hernia Database recommendations for the management of inguinal and femoral hernia in adults. Dan Med Bull. 2011;58(2):C4243.

18. Daes J. The enhanced view-totally extraperitoneal technique for repair of inguinal hernia. Surg Endosc. 2012;26(4):1187–9.
19. Köckerling F, Bittner R, Jacob DA, et al. TEP versus TAPP: comparison of the perioperative outcome in 17,587 patients with a primary unilateral inguinal hernia. Surg Endosc. 2015;29(12):3750–60.
20. Wei K, Lu C, Ge L, et al. Different types of mesh fixation for laparoscopic repair of inguinal hernia: a protocol for systematic review and network meta-analysis with randomized controlled trials. Medicine (Baltimore). 2018;97(16):e0423.
21. Deeken CR, Lake SP. Mechanical properties of the abdominal wall and biomaterials utilized for hernia repair. J Mech Behav Biomed Mater. 2017;74:411–27.
22. Gillion JF, Sanders D, Miserez M, Muysoms F. The economic burden of incisional ventral hernia repair: a multicentric cost analysis. Hernia. 2016;20(6):819–30.
23. Ventral Hernia Working Group, Breuing K, Butler CE, et al. Incisional ventral hernias: review of the literature and recommendations regarding the grading and technique of repair. Surgery. 2010;148(3):544–58.
24. Saiding Q, Chen Y, Wang J, et al. Abdominal wall hernia repair: from prosthetic meshes to smart materials. Mater Today Bio. 2023;21:100691.

Bariatric Surgery in the Elderly

20

Ludovico Docimo and Salvatore Tolone

20.1 Introduction

Obesity is currently acknowledged as one of the most significant health challenges worldwide, with a dramatic impact on comorbidity, mortality, and quality of life (QoL). Metabolic and bariatric surgery (MBS) was traditionally considered inappropriate for elderly patients due to perceived elevated risks, limited physiological reserve, and reduced life expectancy. However, the increasing prevalence of obesity in patients aged 65 years and older, combined with advances in surgical techniques, anesthesia, and perioperative care, has led to a fundamental reassessment of this assumption. Also, the restriction imposed by birthdate rather than by the evaluation of a "biological" age is an outdated concept that can limit access to MBS for patients who are fit for surgery. Recent evidence-based guidelines jointly produced by the American Society for Metabolic and Bariatric Surgery (ASMBS) and the International Federation for the Surgery of Obesity and Metabolic Disorders (IFSO) explicitly state that there is no upper age limit for MBS; rather, candidacy should be determined by individualized assessment with emphasis on comorbidities and frailty rather than chronological age [1].

The purpose of this chapter is to provide a comprehensive and critical review of MBS in elderly patients, focusing on patient selection, the role of frailty, procedure selection (sleeve gastrectomy [SG], Roux-en-Y gastric bypass [RYGB], one-anastomosis gastric bypass [OAGB], and malabsorptive operations), perioperative risk, weight and metabolic outcomes, revisional surgery, nutritional management, and future perspectives.

L. Docimo · S. Tolone (✉)
General, Mininvasive, Oncological and Bariatric Surgery Unit, University of Campania Luigi Vanvitelli, Naples, Italy
e-mail: ludovico.docimo@unicampania.it; salvatore.tolone@unicampania.it

P. Carcoforo, F. Catena (eds.), *Geriatric Surgery*, Updates in Surgery,
https://doi.org/10.1007/978-3-032-24281-5_20

20.2 Epidemiology and Rationale for Metabolic and Bariatric Surgery in the Elderly

The demographic shift toward an aging population intersects with the continuing rise in obesity. In the United States, recent estimates indicate that approximately 41% of individuals aged 65–74 years and nearly 28% of those over 75 years are classified as subjects with obesity; similar trends are observed across Europe, and while baseline prevalence is lower in many Asian countries, it has risen sharply over the past two decades [2]. By 2050, nearly one in three residents in many developed countries will be ≥65 years old, expanding the pool of older adults living with obesity and its sequelae [2]. From a geriatric medicine standpoint, obesity accelerates sarcopenia and functional decline, increases the incidence and severity of osteoarthritis and chronic pain, and it is associated with cardiometabolic diseases, including type 2 diabetes mellitus (T2DM), hypertension, dyslipidemia, atherosclerotic cardiovascular disease, and obstructive sleep apnea syndrome (OSAS) [3–5].

Robust evidence now supports the rationale for offering MBS to older adults. A 14-study systematic review including 3923 septuagenarians reported a mean excess weight loss (EWL) of 54.7% at one year; postoperative major morbidity and mortality were reported to be ~2% and ~1%, respectively. Thus, laparoscopic MBS can be considered effective and acceptably safe even in patients ≥70 years [2]. Complementary national and multicenter data in patients ≥65 years showed clinically relevant reductions in T2DM, blood pressure normalization, and reduced OSAS severity scores after MBS, with a linear improvement in mobility and autonomy with daily activities [3, 4]. Taken together, these data argue that in the elderly, the goals of MBS extend beyond weight reduction to include remission of comorbidities, restoration of daily activities, maintenance of autonomy, and reduction of pharmacological therapy as well as reduction of national healthcare expenses.

20.3 Patient Selection and Preoperative Evaluation

Selection for MBS in older adults must center on the patient's biological rather than chronological age. Frailty—defined as a state of decreased physiologic reserve and increased vulnerability to stressors—is a key determinant of outcomes. Validated tools such as the Clinical Frailty Scale and the Edmonton Frail Scale should be integrated into routine assessment. In a contemporary cohort analysis of laparoscopic sleeve gastrectomy (LSG), Bekhor et al. found that frailty was associated with significantly higher rates of perioperative complications (Clavien-Dindo grade III/IV 8% vs. 3% in non-frail patients) and lower weight-loss effectiveness at 6, 12, and 24 months; notably, age alone was not an independent predictor of safety or efficacy [6].

Beyond frailty, specific predictors of success have been identified in elderly populations. In a multicenter cohort (n = 274) of patients >65 years, Karpińska et al. observed that higher preoperative BMI (per-unit odds ratio [OR] ≈0.90 for achieving >50% EWL), shorter T2DM duration (≤10 years; OR ≈0.30 for failure when

>10 years), and undergoing OAGB (OR ≈15.7 for success) were independently associated with weight-loss success one year post-surgery; conversely, greater preoperative weight loss and longer time since first visit were negatively associated with achieving >50% EWL, perhaps reflecting selection and behavioral confounders [7]. These findings underscore the importance of individualized, data-informed counseling that aligns patient goals with procedure selection and realistic expectations.

Preoperative workup in older adults should include: comprehensive cardiopulmonary evaluation (with echocardiography or stress testing when indicated), sleep apnea assessment, nutritional evaluation (including micronutrients and sarcopenia screening), bone health assessment, and cognitive and psychosocial screening. Optimization of glycemic control and blood pressure, smoking cessation, thromboprophylaxis planning, and prehabilitation (targeted exercise and protein optimization) are recommended best practices. Guidelines emphasize multidisciplinary decision-making and shared goal-setting with patients and caregivers [1, 8].

20.4 Surgical Procedures and Technical Considerations

Procedure choice in the elderly requires balancing perioperative safety and long-term efficacy, as well as considering reflux disease, nutritional risk, and the feasibility of adherence to supplementation. Across international surveys, most bariatric surgeons prefer LSG as the primary operation for patients >65 years, largely owing to its technical simplicity, shorter operative times, and lower perioperative complication rates [9]. However, high-quality comparative data provide important nuance.

Randomized and prospective data: In a randomized study of patients >65 years (BASE trial program and 3-year extension), Pajecki and colleagues found that RYGB produced substantially greater total weight loss (TWL) and EWL than LSG at 3 years (%TWL 30.3% vs. 17.2%; %EWL 63.1% vs. 43.5%), with superior improvements in HbA_{1c}, HDL, LDL, and triglycerides after RYGB; yet adherence to micronutrient supplementation was paradoxically higher after LSG (72% vs. 22%), and parathyroid hormone levels rose more after RYGB, reflecting higher long-term nutritional demands [10, 11]. These findings illustrate the classic trade-off in the elderly: RYGB offers stronger metabolic efficacy but requires rigorous supplementation and surveillance.

Sleeve vs. bypass in older adults—umbrella meta-analysis: Complementing trial data, an umbrella review synthesizing meta-analyses in patients ≥60 years reported that LSG was associated with markedly lower early- and late-emerging complication risks than RYGB (≈55% and 41% relative reductions), whereas RYGB achieved greater EWL by ~15 percentage points and tended to confer greater remission of hypertension and OSAS; T2DM remission nuances favored SG by a small margin in pooled analyses, reflecting heterogeneity in baseline diabetes severity and follow-up [12].

OAGB: In elderly cohorts, OAGB has shown promising results. In a national multicenter study of patients ≥65 years (n = 284), OAGB outperformed LSG and

RYGB for weight loss in adjusted comparisons (higher %EWL and %TWL), and contributed to remission or improvement of T2DM in ~64% and hypertension in ~46% overall; LSG was the most common operation (82%) in that study, reflecting real-world surgeon preference, whereas OAGB appeared metabolically potent despite lower utilization [3]. Karpińska et al. further identified OAGB as an independent predictor of success at one year in older adults [7].

Malabsorptive procedures (biliopancreatic diversion with a duodenal switch [BPD/DS]): Classic malabsorptive procedures remain rarely indicated in elderly patients because of heightened risks of protein-calorie malnutrition, vitamin deficiencies, and bone disease. While they can deliver exceptional weight loss and T2DM remission in selected individuals, careful risk-benefit appraisal is essential, and long-term adherence to intensive supplementation is mandatory—barriers that are often magnified with aging.

Technical pearls in geriatric MBS: Older patients more frequently harbor large hiatal hernias and long-standing gastroesophageal reflux syndrome (GERD); this should influence the choice toward RYGB when reflux is prominent or when esophagitis/Barrett's esophagus is present. Prior abdominal operations are common; dense adhesions increase operative complexity. Prudent trocar placement, careful tissue handling (given increased tissue fragility), and liberal use of energy devices and hemostatic adjuncts can reduce bleeding risk—an important point given that intraperitoneal hemorrhage is the single most common complication reported in cohorts >65 years [5].

20.5 Perioperative Morbidity and Mortality

Multiple contemporary analyses confirm that MBS in carefully selected elderly patients is associated with low perioperative mortality and acceptable morbidity. In a systematic review focused on patients ≥70 years (14 retrospective studies; 3923 patients), pooled major morbidity and mortality were ~2% and ~1%, respectively [2]. In a multicenter cohort of 284 Polish patients ≥65 years undergoing laparoscopic MBS between 2008 and 2022, the overall complication rate was 7.0% (n = 20), the most frequent being intraperitoneal bleeding (2.8%); notably, there was no postoperative mortality reported, and mean follow-up was 47.5 months [5]. On multivariable analysis, longer length of stay and greater %EWL were associated with increased odds of general complications (OR ≈1.17 and 1.02 per unit, respectively), whereas greater preoperative weight loss reduced hemorrhagic complications (OR ≈0.89), and longer length of stay was linked to anastomotic leak (OR ≈1.18) [5].

Large database evaluations reinforce these findings but also highlight age-related gradients in risk. Using the 2022 Metabolic and Bariatric Surgery Accreditation and Quality Improvement Program (MBSAQIP), Ghodasara et al. compared SG outcomes across pediatric, adult, and elderly cohorts and found that, while weight reduction at 30 days was meaningful across all groups, the elderly cohort experienced higher rates of mortality and complications, including sepsis, reoperation, and readmission, reflecting higher preoperative comorbidity burdens (e.g., OSAS, GERD, hypertension) [13]. Importantly, minimally invasive approaches confer significant advantages in older adults: pooled data show reduced pulmonary complications, fewer wound problems, and shorter length of stay compared with open operations [2]. Enhanced Recovery After Surgery (ERAS®) elements—multimodal, opioid-sparing analgesia; goal-directed fluids; early mobilization; and standardized pathways—appear particularly beneficial in the elderly and should be considered standard of care.

20.6 Weight Loss and Metabolic Outcomes

Weight reduction in the elderly after MBS is substantial and durable, albeit often slightly less pronounced than in younger adults—differences that do not diminish clinical value. In the multicenter Polish series of ≥65-year-olds, mean %EWL was ~50.9% and %TWL ~20.6% at long-term follow-up, with significant improvements in comorbidities: among those with T2DM at baseline, 63.7% achieved complete or partial remission; among those with hypertension, 45.9% achieved complete or partial remission [3]. These real-world outcomes are consistent with the broader septuagenarian meta-analytic estimate of ~54.7% EWL at one year [2].

Procedure-specific differences are clinically important. In the elderly randomized trial by Pajecki et al., RYGB outperformed LSG at three years not only for weight loss (%EWL 63.1% vs. 43.5%) but also for glycemic control (HbA_{1c} reduction) and lipid parameters (increases in HDL; decreases in LDL and triglycerides) [10]. An umbrella synthesis of meta-analyses in older adults similarly found that RYGB achieved greater EWL (+~15 percentage points) and offered advantages in hypertension and OSAS remission, whereas LSG had lower early and late complication risks and slightly favored T2DM remission in pooled models [12]. Taken together, these data suggest that in older diabetics with significant reflux or dyslipidemia, RYGB may be the metabolically stronger option—provided that the patient can adhere to the greater nutritional demands of a bypass.

Single-center experiences reinforce the magnitude of benefit. In a retrospective series of 103 elderly patients, Kachmar et al. reported mean %EWL of 31.9%, 43.7%, and 53.4% at 3, 6, and 12 months, respectively, with no 30-day mortality; although the one-year EWL was statistically lower than pooled outcomes reported in non-elderly adults (e.g., historical meta-analysis), it was comparable to elderly-focused meta-analytic estimates, underscoring consistent real-world effectiveness in geriatric populations [4, 14].

20.7 Impact on Comorbidities, Quality of Life, and Functional Status

The benefits of MBS in elderly patients extend beyond weight metrics to meaningful improvements in disease burden, functional capacity, and QoL. Across studies, reductions in antihypertensive and antidiabetic medications are common; OSAS severity decreases with weight loss, improving sleep quality and daytime functioning; osteoarthritis-related pain abates with reduced mechanical load, enabling greater physical activity and independence. While standardized QoL instruments specific to geriatric bariatric patients are not universally applied, global tools such as the Short Form-36 Health Survey (SF-36) and bariatric tools like the Bariatric Analysis and Reporting Outcome System (BAROS) typically show significant gains in physical functioning, vitality, and general health perceptions after surgery.

In revisional cohorts, improvements in QoL are also evident. In a five-year follow-up of elderly patients undergoing revisional bariatric surgery after restrictive operations (e.g., adjustable gastric banding [AGB], SG), Abu-Abeid et al. reported mean BMI ~29.2 and total weight loss ~20.3%, with significant reductions in the prevalence of associated medical problems at last follow-up; early major complication rates were acceptable (4.3% after prior banding and 12.5% after prior sleeve), and readmission was higher in the prior-sleeve subgroup, reflecting the complexity of reflux and sleeve-related issues [15]. These data indicate that carefully selected revisional procedures can restore effectiveness and improve symptoms and QoL in older adults.

20.8 Nutritional Aspects and Long-term Surveillance

Older adults are particularly vulnerable to macro- and micronutrient deficiencies before and after MBS. Age-related anorexia, sarcopenia, diminished gastric acid secretion, polypharmacy (e.g., metformin, proton-pump inhibitors, and chronic inflammation can coexist with obesity to produce baseline deficiencies in vitamin D, iron, and B12. Postoperatively, all procedures reduce intake, while bypass operations add malabsorption of iron, calcium, and fat-soluble vitamins. ASMBS guidelines recommend lifelong supplementation (e.g., daily multivitamin with minerals; additional elemental iron with vitamin C; calcium citrate with vitamin D; vitamin B12 by oral high-dose or parenteral routes as needed) and periodic laboratory surveillance (complete blood count, iron studies, B12, folate, 25-OH vitamin D, calcium, parathyroid hormone), with bone density monitoring and specific attention to protein intake (≥60–80 g/day, individualized higher targets in sarcopenia) [8].

The randomized data in older adults highlight these issues: in Pajecki et al., adherence to supplementation was substantially higher after LSG than after RYGB (72% vs. 22%), and parathyroid hormone increased over time—particularly in bypass patients—despite overall stable hemoglobin and albumin levels [10]. These findings emphasize two practical points in geriatric care: (1) shared decision-making should explicitly weigh long-term nutritional complexity when choosing a bypass procedure; and (2) structured follow-up, patient education, and caregiver engagement are essential to sustain adherence and prevent deficiency-related complications (anemia, neuropathy, osteopenia/osteoporosis). Telemedicine touchpoints, automated reminders, and coordination with primary care/geriatrics may improve adherence in older adults.

20.9 Revisional Bariatric Surgery in the Elderly

With increasing longevity after primary MBS and with many elderly patients bearing a history of legacy restrictive operations (AGB, vertical banded gastroplasty [VBG]), the need for revisional or conversional procedures has grown. Revisional surgery in older adults can address weight regain, inadequate weight loss, refractory GERD, band erosion/slippage, or sleeve-related complications. At a specialized center, Abu-Abeid et al. reported acceptable early major complication rates (4–13%), durable TWL of ~20%, and significant reduction of associated medical problems over a median ~5 years, supporting feasibility in carefully selected elderly patients [15].

National registry analyses clarify risk profiles by conversion type. Using MBSAQIP 2020–2022, Barajas-Gamboa et al. identified 3746 elderly patients undergoing conversional MBS among 51,138 total conversions. Primary AGB (55.6% of elderly conversions) most commonly converted to LSG (57.6%) or RYGB (39.7%); VBG (4.8%) was converted to RYGB in 92.8%. Notably, conversions from AGB to RYGB had higher rates of serious complications and death (7.9% and 0.7%) than conversions to other techniques. VBG to RYGB exhibited the highest morbidity (18.4%) and mortality (4.1%), likely reflecting operative complexity and comorbidity accrual, although comparisons were limited by small sample sizes [16]. These patterns suggest that, in elderly patients requiring conversion, careful selection of target procedure (e.g., avoiding high-risk VBG→RYGB when suitable alternatives exist) and meticulous perioperative optimization are paramount.

20.10 Frailty, Functional Reserve, and Prehabilitation

Frailty is a multidimensional construct encompassing weakness, exhaustion, slowed performance, low activity, and unintentional weight loss; it correlates with adverse outcomes across surgical disciplines. In geriatric bariatric surgery, frailty stratifies risk more meaningfully than age. Bekhor et al. found that frailty predicted both safety (higher severe complication rates) and effectiveness (lower %EWL and treatment success across two years) after LSG, whereas chronological age did not independently alter outcomes [6]. Pragmatically, routine frailty screening (Clinical Frailty Scale, Edmonton Frail Scale) should inform shared decisions about procedure type, venue (high-acuity centers), postoperative monitoring intensity, and the need for prehabilitation.

Prehabilitation bundles—progressive resistance and aerobic exercise, protein optimization (with leucine-rich supplements), vitamin D repletion, smoking cessation, respiratory training, and medication review to deprescribe sedatives—may bolster physiologic reserve. Although randomized evidence tailored to elderly MBS is limited, geriatric surgery literature suggests improvements in functional capacity and reductions in pulmonary complications with prehabilitation.

Integrating these elements into bariatric pathways for older adults is a reasonable best practice.

20.11 Future Perspectives and Evolving Therapeutic Algorithms

Rapid progress in anti-obesity pharmacotherapy—glucagon-like peptide-1 receptor agonists (GLP-1 RAs) and dual incretin agonists—creates new opportunities for staged or combined approaches in elderly patients. In an international survey of 184 bariatric surgeons across 53 countries, Dowgiałło-Gornowicz et al. reported that 77% prescribe anti-obesity medications, with a consensus to prefer pharmacotherapy in older adults with BMI 30–35 kg/m^2 and to use medications perioperatively to optimize high-BMI patients prior to surgery; LSG was the most commonly preferred primary operation in those >65 years [9]. Such hybrid models may reduce perioperative risk (via preoperative weight loss), improve metabolic status, and support maintenance post-surgery.

Technological and systems innovations are also pertinent. Robotic assistance and refined energy devices may further reduce bleeding and conversions to open surgery in complex elderly cases. Standardized ERAS® protocols tailored to geriatric physiology, enhanced telemedicine follow-up, and integration with primary care and geriatrics for long-term nutritional surveillance can address adherence gaps highlighted in randomized elderly cohorts [8, 10]. Finally, future research priorities include randomized trials explicitly enrolling patients ≥70 years, head-to-head comparisons of RYGB vs OAGB in elderly diabetics with reflux, and long-term endpoints encompassing functional independence, frailty trajectories, cognition, and cost-effectiveness.

20.12 Conclusions

In contemporary practice, MBS is a valuable and increasingly indispensable option for selected elderly patients living with obesity. Safety is acceptable when care is delivered in experienced centers and guided by frailty-aware selection and optimization. LSG offers a favorable perioperative profile, whereas RYGB (and in some series OAGB) confers stronger long-term metabolic efficacy—particularly in patients with T2DM and GERD—at the cost of greater nutritional surveillance. Revisional procedures can restore efficacy but carry higher risk; national registry data provide procedure-specific guidance. Across the evidence base, the organizing principle is clear: biological age, frailty status, and patient goals—not chronological age—should guide decision-making. With population aging, MBS will play an expanding role in prolonging healthy life expectancy, reducing polypharmacy and disease burden, and improving quality of life in older adults.

References

1. De Luca M, Shikora S, Eisenberg D, et al. Scientific evidence for the updated guidelines on indications for metabolic and bariatric surgery (IFSO/ASMBS). Obes Surg. 2024;34(11):3963–4096.
2. Kapała J, Maroszczuk T, Dowgiałło-Gornowicz N. Efficacy and safety of laparoscopic bariatric surgery in patients of 70 years and older: a systematic review and meta-analysis. Obes Rev. 2025;26(3):e13867.
3. Dowgiałło-Gornowicz N, Lech P, Major P, Collaborative Study Group. Bariatric and metabolic surgery in patients older than 65 years – a multicenter study. Obes Surg. 2023;33(10):3106–11.
4. Kachmar M, Soliman I, Mason N, et al. Bariatric surgery in the elderly population: a multi-surgeon, single-institution retrospective review. JSLS. 2023;27(3):e2023.00028.
5. Dowgiałło-Gornowicz N, Lech P, Katkowski B, et al. Risk factors for bariatric surgery in patients over 65 years of age – a multicenter retrospective cohort study. Langenbecks Arch Surg. 2024;409(1):115.
6. Bekhor EY, Kirshtein B, Peleg N, et al. Frailty Index as a predictor of operative safety and efficacy in patients undergoing laparoscopic sleeve gastrectomy. Obes Surg. 2025;35(5):1603–10.
7. Karpińska I, Dowgiałło-Gornowicz N, Franczak P, et al. Factors contributing to weight loss success after bariatric procedures in patients over 65 years old: a multicenter retrospective cohort study. Int J Surg. 2024;110(8):4893–9.
8. Mechanick JI, Apovian C, Brethauer S, et al. Clinical Practice Guidelines for the perioperative nutrition, metabolic, and nonsurgical support of patients undergoing bariatric procedures – 2019 update: cosponsored by American Association of Clinical Endocrinologists/American College of Endocrinology, The Obesity Society, American Society for Metabolic & Bariatric Surgery, Obesity Medicine Association, and American Society of Anesthesiologists. Surg Obes Relat Dis. 2020;16(2):175–247.
9. Dowgiałło-Gornowicz N, Wityk M, Jaworski P, et al. Obesity solutions for patients over 65 years of age: surgeon perspectives on anti-obesity medications and metabolic bariatric surgery – International survey study. Obes Surg. 2025;35(8):3182–9.
10. Pajecki D, Dos Anjos Pinheiro MC, Dantas ACB, et al. Sleeve gastrectomy versus Roux-en-Y gastric bypass for treating obesity in patients >65 years old: 3-year outcomes of a randomized trial. J Gastrointest Surg. 2023;27(4):780–2.
11. Pajecki D, Dantas ACB, Kanaji AL, et al. Bariatric surgery in the elderly: randomized prospective study comparing safety of sleeve gastrectomy and Roux-en-Y gastric bypass (BASE Trial). Surg Obes Relat Dis. 2020;16(10):1436–40.
12. Kermansaravi M, Vitiello A, Valizadeh R, et al. Comparing the safety and efficacy of sleeve gastrectomy versus Roux-en-Y gastric bypass in elderly (>60 years) with severe obesity: an umbrella systematic review and meta-analysis. Int J Surg. 2023;109(11):3541–50.
13. Ghodasara SK, Elsawwah JK, Yang HJ, et al. Clinical outcomes of varying age groups following vertical sleeve gastrectomy: a retrospective study using the 2022 MBSAQIP database in the United States. J Minim Invasive Surg. 2025;28(2):89–96.
14. Buchwald H, Avidor Y, Braunwald E, et al. Bariatric surgery: a systematic review and meta-analysis. JAMA. 2004;292(14):1724–37.
15. Abu-Abeid A, Gosher N, Shnell M, et al. Revision of restrictive bariatric procedures in elderly patients: results at a 5-year follow-up. Updates Surg. 2024;76(8):2825–31.
16. Barajas-Gamboa JS, Restrepo-Rodas G, Mocanu V, et al. Evaluating postoperative conversion trends in the elderly: an Metabolic and Bariatric Surgery Accreditation and Quality Improvement Program-based analysis of bariatric surgery outcomes. Surg Obes Relat Dis. 2025;21(8):949–55.

GPSR Compliance

The European Union's (EU) General Product Safety Regulation (GPSR) is a set of rules that requires consumer products to be safe and our obligations to ensure this.

If you have any concerns about our products, you can contact us on ProductSafety@springernature.com

In case Publisher is established outside the EU, the EU authorized representative is:

Springer Nature Customer Service Center GmbH
Europaplatz 3
69115 Heidelberg, Germany

Printed by Wilco bv, the Netherlands